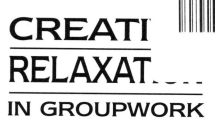

CREATIVE
RELAXATION
IN GROUPWORK

Dedication

This book is dedicated to my loving parents, Arthur and Margaret Sherwin, and to my dear mother-in-law, Nell Tubbs, who through her suffering re-emphasized for me the importance of using relaxation and stress management techniques to cope with life.

CREATIVE
RELAXATION
IN GROUPWORK

Irene Tubbs

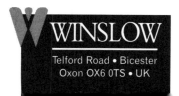

WINSLOW

Telford Road • Bicester
Oxon OX6 0TS • UK

First published in 1996 by
Winslow Press Ltd, Telford Road, Bicester, Oxon OX6 0TS, United Kingdom
Reprinted 1997

© Irene Tubbs, 1996

002-2286 Printed in Great Britain (HtP)

British Library Cataloguing in Publication Data
Tubbs, Irene
Creative relaxation in groupwork
  1. Relaxation 2. Relaxation — Therapeutic use
  I. Title
  615.8'51

ISBN 0 86388 143 2

CONTENTS

IRENE TUBBS has been working in the field of education since 1976, initially as a physical education specialist working with children and adults. In 1978 she was a founder–contributor of a rehabilitation programme set up to assist patients recovering from any condition that affects the heart, a programme which she still offers.

In 1984 she became a senior lecturer in adult education, and was subsequently a head of department and then a head of area, being an initiator of many educational courses for all age groups. As well as performing a management role, she also continued to organize and run courses for trainers and students in coronary rehabilitation, relaxation, stress management, diet/nutrition, benefits of exercise, fertility counselling, appraisal and management skills. She has previously written books on coronary rehabilitation and fertility, plus many pamphlets and self-help guidelines for combating stress.

As well as a teaching degree, Irene has diplomas in management, counselling, stress management, multi-modal psychotherapy and stress counselling.

FOREWORD

Relaxation has long been recognized as being of significant benefit to individuals. In this book Irene Tubbs has put together a variety of techniques aimed at a wide client group found in many types of 'helping' situations.

Practitioners of counselling, cognitive–behavioural psycho-therapy and stress counselling have been using relaxation as a way of helping clients for many years. The use of relaxation amongst those undergoing infertility treatment has also proved beneficial.

There is much in this book to recommend it both to the beginner and to the seasoned practitioner. In addition to the areas indicated above, it examines the benefits of human touch and the role relaxation plays in creating the most helpful type of environment. This useful publication will add to the body of practical knowledge on the subject.

GLADEANA McMAHON
Co-director, counselling and psychotherapy courses
Centre for Stress Management, London

ACKNOWLEDGEMENTS

It is within one's own family that the beginnings of understanding and dealing with life are formulated. This understanding is born of love, care and attention, all of which I have received and given. To all my family I say thank you for the pleasure of being part of your lives and for supporting me in my endeavours to help others.

Throughout my working life my pupils, students and colleagues have contributed greatly to my exploration and development, and to the beliefs I hold. In particular I am indebted to my coronary groups, whose tenacity in dealing with illness and stress has given me the impetus to devise self-help processes for change that are manageable for individuals.

INTRODUCTION

Through the ages many different methods have been used to try to reach a state of relaxation, either to reduce physical and emotional symptoms of stress or to enhance an individual's capacity to deal with pressure. The word 'relaxation' itself has many connotations, depending on the needs, desires and pressures of a particular society. These pressures influence and spring from our very existence. They encourage inventiveness, spur us on and promote self-evaluation. Pressure therefore has a positive side that can be enhanced by the use of relaxation techniques, but it is when pressure threatens to create unmanageable levels of stress that those techniques are most effective. The most beneficial way of reducing stress is to use relaxation techniques not only as an entity in their own right, but also as a foundation upon which to build emotional and physical coping skills within other techniques.

Throughout this book, you will be made aware of the many different possibilities for reducing stress and managing pressure, the aim being to provide self-help coping strategies that create feelings of self-control. Manageable and unmanageable levels of stress are dealt with in greater detail under 'Stress Management' in Section 2. You will be able to reflect on a variety of techniques and their processes whose aim is either to help to relax the mind, to work primarily on the body, to promote body and mind/spirit harmony, to focus on complete muscular relaxation, to promote concentration or to increase sensory awareness.

All the therapies recognize the healing capacity within us and strive to encourage its release by practical application. As you will see, this book favours a 'body and mind' approach whose processes have a 'stepping stone' application to relaxation. This process is seen as a progressive means of learning that is perceived by the individual as attainable: small increments of success that stimulate greater interest and awareness.

The aim throughout this book is to engender an interest in readers to explore for themselves and within groupwork the many different ways of achieving relaxation, with the emphasis on feeling good and being in control. My ultimate goal was to provide a resource that contained many different avenues of exploration, highlighting my own expertise and the expertise of others. This book is meant, not as a 'Gospel' approach to, but as a means of, exploration, practice and change. It is clearly written both for practitioners in the field, as a means of reinforcing their beliefs while encouraging thoughts on other avenues, and for those who are just beginning to work in this field or wish to do so in the future.

We have a clients' market, with many different approaches and styles from which to choose. The practitioner's role, I believe, is to encourage participants to learn the basics of relaxation through training and then to recognize that they have the freedom to choose avenues of enhancement for the future. A list of alternative therapies is therefore provided in the appendix for the reader's consideration.

This book is in four sections. *Section 1* deals with evidence of the benefits of relaxation and *Section 2* with the actual theoretical and practical methods of relaxation. *Section 3* provides constructive guidelines for good practice. *Section 4*, the core of the book, comprises actual workshop practice, upon which readers may base and develop their ideas. The appendix provides information on alternative therapies, relevant reading matter and visual aids.

THE BENEFITS OF RELAXATION

The evidence surrounding relaxation and its benefits

The word 'relaxation' has several meanings (I later detail words you could use with your clients) but for most people it means 'feeling good'. It can be used any time, anywhere, in any situation in order to restore a sense of self-control, even if only momentary. Its main purpose is to reduce negative physiological and emotional feelings through the release of tension, the restoring of energy and the encouragement of calming thought processes. The benefits can be felt when relaxation is practised intermittently but its greatest effect will be felt and maintained if practice becomes part of our everyday lives, an automatic process, triggered whenever we recognize aspects of our physical or emotional well-being that give us a feeling of not being in control. Relaxation is thus a way of counterbalancing our levels of stress, becoming second nature as with an athlete who trains or a typist who learns a keyboard.

The opposite state to relaxation is *tension* often accompanied by anxiety. At some stage a whole range of *physical, emotional and behavioural* effects can be felt, as well as effects on *logical thinking*. For example: abnormal posture, neckache, backache, headache, restlessness, nausea, tiredness, stiffness, sleeplessness, agitation, anxiety, low self-esteem. One way for individuals to understand tension is to see it as a piece of elastic. When tense it is stretched tight, rigid, inflexible; when loose it is firm but stretchable.

How then does relaxation help? Let us look at the evidence.

1 It acts as a safety valve, to release and relieve tension effectively.
2 It reduces our stress response to situations.
3 It relieves aching muscles.
4 It reduces pain, such as neckache or backache, by releasing tension.
5 It reduces fatigue by helping us not to waste energy, enabling a quicker recovery after effort, as it recharges our internal 'batteries'.
6 It promotes sleep, by clearing the mind of everyday thoughts, and enhances our learning capabilities by clearing the mind of non-productive thoughts.
7 It can help to improve personal relationships because we can be calmer and more rational.
8 It gives one the feeling of well-being.
9 Where tension can increase the physical level of pain we are experiencing, relaxation actually reduces it.

10 If we are able to relax at will, tension will drop and be replaced by calmness, control, confidence and more energy to put to good use.

11 Relaxation gives us time for ourselves, to concentrate on our own well-being, shutting out everything else that is going on around us.

12 It provides an opportunity for us to regain control in a situation where our anxiety levels are high and we can begin to feel out of control.

13 It enhances our natural coping skills and acts as an enabling process for dealing with problems.

14 It increases our social skills: making friends is easier with someone who is relaxed and at ease.

15 It has a physiological effect on the body as the heart rate and breathing slow, releasing hormones into the blood stream, which enhances the feeling of calmness and reduces tension.

16 By voluntarily relaxing our muscles we relax our minds too, so we can feel calmer emotionally as well as physically.

The aims of relaxation therefore are to enable us to identify tension, by being aware of what it feels like, using techniques to alter its physical effect on us; to get rid of that tension by relaxing individual muscles, the whole body and mind; and to provide the ability to use a particular technique at any time or place, whenever we feel the need. This can be of short duration (a few seconds or minutes) or for a longer period of time (half an hour to an hour, or sometimes longer).

Relaxation can be perceived as passive or active. *Passive* when it is controlled by an exterior force without resistance, as with massage, reflexology or aromatherapy, *active* when individuals themselves actively work at relaxing their bodies, as with yoga, exercise, deep breathing, meditation and visualization. As will be seen, there are many techniques that either have a relaxation basis or provide opportunities to relax within another concept.

There is no age barrier where relaxation is concerned. Indeed, the younger we are when we begin to use these techniques the more 'second nature' they become — a natural part of rapidly changing lives — so that children learn to use them to their maximum potential in the same way that they develop their learning of a language or physical prowess. Children who are helped to recognize tension and use a relaxation response can discover their own ways of dealing with stressful times in their lives. As has been so aptly stated by **Jane Madder** in her book, *Relax and Be Happy*

(1987), 'Relaxation involves no drugs, is wholly under the control of the individual and, like the most physical skills, it is best learnt in childhood.'

This leads us on to the recognition of how much better an adolescent will be able to deal with the difficulties of puberty if they have learned a way of dealing with stress. This concept of being in control increases their capacity to learn. Within the educational field it is widely recognized that anxiety acts as a block to understanding. It sets up a poor pattern of self-perception, disrupting efficient learning, with a subsequent lack of interest or fear of failing in a child or adult. For example, when a person is tense this tension will affect their motor/co-ordination skills. Similarly awareness of their bodily changes, that may appear to be different from those of their peers, will often create self-destructive thoughts, heightening feelings of not being in control. Relaxation techniques provide reflection time for them to challenge and deal with these thoughts and strive to replace them with realistic, constructive ones.

Studies have shown that some children are susceptible to severe stress disorders brought on by their inability to deal with emotional or behavioural problems in their school years that can handicap them in their everyday lives. These problems may arise, for example, from social trends that encourage competition and a desire to be the best, without children having the skills to cope with possible failure, so that when they reach adulthood they have difficulty making decisions for themselves for fear of failure, often avoiding a situation rather than dealing with it.

Children often have these confused feelings and thoughts, but workshops can open up avenues that provide the opportunity for them to feel in control. This can be achieved in many ways, but the foundation is often one based on improving their physical skills, as it is a recognized fact that children's self-esteem is very closely linked to physical prowess. This development helps them to feel good about themselves, one of the crowd, not the odd one out. It is also actually *seen* by themselves and others and is proof that they are capable, increasing their confidence to try new skills or improve still further on the ones they have already attained. Such development is also recognized as being particularly helpful for children with hyperactive tendencies, where strenuous activities have allowed them to release their energy and then be prepared for relaxation exercises that enhance their feelings of control, moving from overactivity to underactivity in a positive way. Success breeds the desire for success in children, as it does in adults: they want to learn more and achieve more, but in the process they need to be able to

5

deal with failure — otherwise everything that goes wrong in their lives will be perceived as a major catastrophe.

There is a widely held belief that behavioural traits that are stress-related often have an element of family history that demonstrates an adult's tendency to behave in the same way. Children imitate and watch our every move: if we are prone to angry outbursts, mood swings or depression, our children are likely to follow suit. If we laugh, so will they; if we are seen to relax they will want to join in, too. Remember that body language cannot be hidden!

Where lack of ability to control stress in young lives is continued into adulthood we can see that it exacerbates the effects of the pace at which we live our lives. Life becomes a continual challenge, often with increased pressure and heightened expectations from ourselves and our peers. Time and again in my work with clients we have been able to establish that a particular destructive behavioural trait they use has been learnt in their childhood and, when replaced by an effective relaxation technique, has diminished. Often a technique is linked to a thought-challenging process that enables a physical and emotional change to occur. Sometimes it becomes apparent that individuals have had relaxation skills in the past, but that they have forgotten them or are not using them to help with a particular situation. Adults need more support and encouragement to practise these skills, as destructive avoidance, or pressures of time, can hinder belief in their effectiveness.

It is also apparent that high levels of emotional stress increase our susceptibility to illness, as chronic stress results in a suppression of the immune system, which in turn leads to hormonal imbalances. These imbalances could increase the production of abnormal cells at precisely the time the body is least capable of destroying them. This helps us to understand why, when news of an illness is given to an individual, particularly if it is of a serious nature, they may want to live life 'in the slow lane', which in itself tends to establish negative expectations of death rather than recovery. The benefits of relaxation techniques therefore are enormous, not least since emotion, which is often linked to illness, can also contribute to health. Research has also shown that after illness, when the body is weak, a quicker, sustained recovery has been achieved where individuals use relaxation techniques to enhance the medical aspects of their recovery. Relaxation is seen as a preventive measure reducing tension, pain and fear of further illness. In particular, relaxation offers the opportunity for an individual to release themselves from pain (as participation in a pleasurable activity is known to reduce pain) and gives them time to think about what may have contributed to their illness and to see the benefits of practising positive ways to alleviate these possible causes in the future. Where an individual has a good reason to recover, having goals in life that they want to attain, their recovery outlook improves. One emphasis that I use in my work in the field of coronary rehabilitation is the attainment of 'quality' of life as opposed to 'quantity'. Once you can establish with someone that it is the quality of their day that matters and how good they felt about it, as opposed to the amount they have crammed into it, they tend to develop a different outlook on life and to perceive pleasure where they would normally perceive pressure and stress.

Simonton *et al* in their book, *Getting Well Again* (Bantam, 1991), highlight the benefits of using relaxation, exercise and visualization alongside traditional medicine in the fight against cancer. They use the concept of various techniques in order to enhance a person's own belief in themselves and their recovery, aiming to provide their patients with personal control over their illness. They particularly believe that 'emotional and mental states play a significant role both in susceptibility to disease, including cancer, and in recovery from all disease'. Basically theirs is an effective treatment programme dealing with the whole person. Anyone who is contemplating working with individuals or groups who are recovering from illness would find the ideas in this book very enlightening and a basis upon which to work.

Edmund Jacobson, whom many perceive as the founder of our present-day beliefs about tension, found during research on people who were reporting anxiety that tension caused muscle fibres to shorten. His initial concept, in 1938, involved tensing and releasing 15 muscle groups, taking 56 one-hour sessions. Since that time his ideas have been revised, although his principles are still adhered to by many practitioners. Others have used an approach of facing a feared situation and then reversing its tension-related consequences through relaxation practice. I use both ideas. In order to understand how and why the body tenses, I begin by establishing the difference between the states of tension and relaxation. Later I use thought processes to enhance this level of awareness, as a way of dealing with fears while in a relaxed state.

Learning and teaching aids

Young adults and teenagers
With older children you will soon become aware of patterns of behaviour that appear to be set and causing anxiety, especially when you learn to read body language signals. Older children are

more prone to question and seek clarification or proof of the benefits of using relaxation techniques, so as well as games there needs to be a group 'sharing' time set aside for them to express how they felt about a particular session, its outcome and its benefits to them. This is particularly helpful for other children in the group who may not have been fully aware of what their feelings were or who were afraid they were not 'normal'.

For example, a workshop on recognizing tension in fingers particularly when studying could involve each individual clasping and releasing an object, feeling the difference between firm and light touch, and recognizing the colour of the fingers when gripping tightly or loosely, followed by discussion of the differences felt by individuals and which is preferable. The workshop could then establish the physiological facts of circulation within the body, how it is hindered by tension and stimulated by effective breathing and exercise techniques. Practice of these techniques encourages circulation to return while highlighting the benefits of doing so when writing.

With teenagers, a workshop based on 'looking good' is often a useful way to demonstrate tension and ways of releasing it. Body language is the key here: teenagers are often very good at demonstrating what they consider to be the 'body message' of another person they either like or find funny. They should not use as an example someone else in the group, but should be asked to think of someone they knew outside school, on the television and so on. The purpose is to establish what is good and bad posture, and what are their benefits and detriments for the way they feel about themselves and others.

Adults
With adults there are many workshop ideas you can use, as you will see in detail later. However, it is important to recognize the need for discussion at the beginning and end of a session relating to the group's feelings about relaxation and its benefits.

Where your workshop is for people recovering from illness, you need to recognize that the majority of them will have a basic concept, even an expectation, that the doctor can provide the remedy to 'cure' their illness. Therefore working with some people to show how much control they can have in their progress may be slow and needs to include evidence of the part they have played and are still playing in their own recovery; for example, in coronary rehabilitation, I take my group through a series of 10 sessions that look at aspects of their illness and ways they can cope with it, together with practical and theoretical benefits of exercise which is progressively increased from 30 minutes to one and a half hours.

1 The heart and how it functions.
2 The importance of breathing techniques to enhance the working of the heart, reduce stress, provide energy and make exercise feel easier.
3 The importance of relaxation techniques in coping with pain and stress, restoring energy levels, promoting positive realistic thoughts and feeling good.
4 Problems associated with illness and practical ways of coping with them.
5 How to consult a doctor (a high stress factor) and ensure medication is taken properly.
6 Diet and its contribution to recovery after illness, as well as simple ways of reducing weight.
7 Stress management: control of pressures in life (many feel stress was a major factor in their illness).
8 Dos and don'ts of exercise (a theory-based reinforcement of the practical exercises we do).
9 Evaluation/clarification of previous sessions, including questions from participants.
10 A full one-and-a-half hour exercise class, followed by 15 minutes' relaxation.

Within every session I also offer the opportunity for each individual to ask questions that I encourage the group to answer.

METHODS OF ACHIEVING RELAXATION

Introduction

This section looks at the possible relaxation methods that can be used, with examples of their implementation and teaching guidelines. It is important to understand our own bodies and, through this understanding, to be able to create an environment that enables other individuals to do the same. I therefore begin this section with exploration of the ways we can and do use body language and our five senses to enhance a relaxed state, before I describe my own breathing and relaxation techniques.

Body language

Across all social groups we can experience agreement or apprehension according to the unspoken messages we believe are being relayed by others. Often our body language is the first clue to our character and personality. Meeting someone for the first time can be a daunting experience; first impressions can trigger instant like or dislike. The key to this first impression is body language, the very basic form of communication. How many times have someone's bodily movements 'put you off them' or, on the contrary, encouraged you to feel comfortable and relaxed? I believe the ability to send the correct messages is a natural prerequisite of every individual and, in a more developed form, a necessary skill of a counsellor or trainer. It is important to recognize that changes in our automatic nervous system occur when we are negative, anxious or angry, and tension is the result. By learning ways of relaxing we can challenge and change these automatic responses.

This section is aimed at heightening *your* awareness of body language in order to enable participants in your workshops to understand their own bodies and use the inner and outer messages in a way that gives them a feeling of being in control. Below are listed common examples of body language. See if you can recognize yourself or other people you know in them.

► Curled up, head down: may denote withdrawal feelings.
► Sitting back, shoulders back, arms open: may denote openness, willingness to listen.
► Nodding, smiling: may denote agreement, attention.
► Eyes raised to ceiling, deep breathing, tight jaw: may denote disagreement, anxiety.
► Eyes down, hands crossed: may denote shyness or guilt.

- Staring, body limp, mouth or jaw drooping: may denote feelings of rejection, sadness.
- Rigid body, arms wrapped around, cowering; may denote fear.
- Frequent sighing, head drooping, shoulders sagging, lack of concentration: may denote depression.
- Tension (rigidity) in neck or shoulders, tight lips: may denote anxiety.
- Hands behind head, body upright: may denote a position of authority.
- Hands behind head, body reclining: may denote lack of interest.
- Sparkling eyes, smiling, open mouth: may denote happiness.
- Head in alignment: may denote confidence.
- Running hands through hair, elbows on desk, head resting on hands: may denote problem-solving mode.
- Stretching, arching back, rubbing body or shoulders: may denote the need to release tension, take a break.
- Stamping feet, shaking arms: may denote frustration, being out of control.
- Tight fists, raised arms, tight muscles, tight jaw, staring eyes: may denote aggressive or defensive mode.
- Defensive body position: may denote unwillingness to listen, resistance to change, refusal to compromise, with thoughts of 'you will not hurt me', 'I am right' demonstrating insecurity.
- Constant eye contact: may mean either that they are trying to dominate or that they are consciously listening to every word that is being said.
- Intermittent eye contact: may denote lack of self-esteem, insecurity,
- Facial expression: may show interest, boredom, cheerfulness, dejection, changing with the way people feel inside or as a means of disguising their true feelings.
- Posture, gesture and touch may be threatening, inviting, defensive or reassuring, depending on the individual, ease or unease. Sympathetic mimicry can help a person to enhance contact, as with counselling.
- Protecting personal space by moving or not responding to the initiations of others may denote a need to withdraw, avoid or protect oneself.
- Grace of children, natural poise: may be lacking if they are suffering emotional upheaval.
- Happy faces exert a calming effect and encourage others to smile; habitually miserable people encourage withdrawal.

No doubt you could add examples of your own.

Teaching and learning aids

Next time you are socializing, travelling in a bus or train, shopping or are involved in any other everyday activity, look around you and watch other people's body language. See if you can ascertain what they are feeling. With family or friends, see if you can detect signals from their bodies which show how they are feeling. Ask them if you are right and whether they have noticed any particular body signals that you tend to display and, if so, what message they think was being conveyed. Just be aware that this is an exercise meant to help you understand your own body language and the body language of others, so that you can help them to understand themselves better. It is not meant as a fault-finding exercise, so the best way to approach it is with humour. Start with yourself. Look at yourself in a mirror, alter your facial features to show different emotions, such as fear, hilarity, amusement, tension and relaxation.

Within the group/client session(s) you will see many different expressions that may signal anxiety. Indeed, some people actively use bodily signals as a means of getting attention and will hold onto them until they can be shown more effective ways to gain the attention they desire. Focusing on understanding body language in a session will enable you to create a comforting environment where openness can be explored. To achieve this I start by demonstrating body language myself, using humour to create a light-hearted atmosphere. This often helps clients to relax.

It is through the ability to interpret body language that an individual will feel able to defuse a situation by changing their bodily messages in order to respond favourably. There is no doubt that the use of body language encourages and enhances friendships — often a reason why people join workshops. When working with individuals or groups you will soon begin to establish that in some situations where individuals have become depressed this has been due to repetitive actions that tend to promote a feeling of tiredness. For example, I have often found that in 'work' situations a client has become depressed because they have remained in a set position for long periods, focusing on their work, often only seeing the problems. Using a system of constructive breaks and breathing exercises, they have been able to break the chain of their negative feelings and tell themselves 'I am in control of what I do', instead of 'My work is in control of me', acquiring a more relaxed approach to their work.

Dr Ida Rolf, a biochemist and physiologist, found that both physical accidents and emotional upsets tightened the muscle tissue and that, if an individual continued to hold the postures of fear, grief or anger for any length of time, these patterns would become set. To help clients or groups to deal with negative body messages that they believe are coming from others, I ask them to visualize themselves at work, seeing the body messages of others and looking at their own. We then discuss this and enact a reversal role-play, where they are encouraged to demonstrate the body message of the 'offending' person and I demonstrate theirs. Once the body language has been established as being correct for both parties, I demonstrate ways of making the body language more open and see if this encourages the other person to do so. This is just a simple way of helping an individual to see if they are misreading the signals or, if we establish that they are not, seeing whether their own body language may be giving off a signal that encourages a negative one back.

Within a group, you need to establish an open forum where each person can demonstrate what they consider to be an offending body message, which can be discussed, evaluated and changed with the group's agreement into one that is positive. From this you can direct your participants to work in pairs or small groups and encourage each person to show what they believe is their body position when they feel slighted by others and actively seek to change it.

It is essential to explore within a group understanding and acceptance of bodily traits that are a necessary part of our genetic and emotional make-up, such as crying, and seeing them as a means of releasing tension. Tears actually contain a natural painkiller called Ankaphalin which helps us to feel better by fighting sorrow and pain. You will find that someone who fights tears because they feel they are a sign of weakness often cries a lot. Accepting that they have a right to cry, perceiving it as natural, reduces the number of times these individuals actually do cry. It is also crucial for them to understand the importance of releasing tension. Within a group, this would be established by discussing how they feel when they are tearful, writing it down and sharing it with others. The sharing opens up their awareness of not being alone, being normal.

Exploration is the key to change

We are all aware that when we laugh we feel relaxed. Laughter is a useful tool for us to demonstrate to others positive ways of releasing tension and establishing a clearer understanding of how the body works. It is crucial that your participants recognize that a relaxed person is likely to live a longer, healthier life, be able to cope better with pain and deal better with others who are not relaxed. Establish what a smile or laughter does for them; help them to see the positive effects (mirrors or partner work can be used here). Laughter lights up the face, makes us look younger, draws people to us, provides rapid relief from tension, opens doors of friendship, encourages acceptance and creates a relaxed atmosphere. French neurologist Henri Rubenstein, who has studied laughter extensively, concludes that one minute of laughter provides up to 45 minutes of relaxation.

Body alignment and posture

As a physical educational specialist I very much endorse the use of body alignment as a promoter of well-being. I am not Alexander-trained (see Appendix) but I do use the theme of good posture as a means of endorsing the process of feeling good. This, linked with understanding body language, will enable your participants to present the posture and deliver the message they wish to.

Teaching and learning aids

Notice how each person sits, stands and interacts. I did this when I was having a break from working on this book, noticing how people in the street carried themselves, some very upright and appearing in control, others slightly bent, looking agitated and tired. What was most interesting is that age made no difference: one woman I would estimate to be about 70 had a wonderful erect posture even though she was carrying some shopping and yet a much younger boy walked with hunched shoulders, hands in pockets, looking down at his feet and narrowly missing walking into a post!

Use everyday occurrences to demonstrate the importance of body messages: for example, courtship, being served in a shop or restaurant, taking a child to school, taking back something that is faulty, breaking something, meeting someone for the first time or learning a new skill.

Encourage an understanding of the clothes and the colours we choose to wear: what messages do they give to us and to others? What messages do we want to give? Are they being received correctly by others?

Our perceptions of good posture are often highlighted when we see good and bad posture in others, such as a model, a gymnast, or a soldier. Take a look at yourself next time you go for a walk and pass a window that reflects your body image. How upright are you? We do this all the time to ensure that what we are wearing looks good, but how much more important it is that it hangs right, so that our appearance is enhanced, not impaired. If we look good we feel good. For many people with depression and anxiety these feelings are based on their dislike of themselves and bits they would like to change.

We can learn so much from observation. It is of crucial importance to a good practitioner and the quality of their practice. Whenever you feel uncomfortable or tense, take stock of the way you are sitting or standing: are you twisted, bent, rigid; where is your head — is it bent forward and down, what sort of alignment does it have with the neck? A useful exercise here is to draw the position your head is in (just use lines) or, more effectively, to get someone else to do it for you. (You can also use this idea in groupwork.) You will be surprised at the position your posture assumes. Certainly as I work at this computer I am constantly aware of a discomfort in my neck and I actively try to re-align my body to reduce this.

If you believe that balance brings good health, vitality and a sense of well-being then you will recognize the importance of looking, listening, asking and feeling in order to develop your own personal awareness of body alignment.

Teenagers and adults

One of the many beliefs I brought to my work as a teacher was the need for the body to be stretched so that it would be able to work harder. Stretching not only means that the muscles can work harder, it also means that the scope of alignment is heightened as the muscles are encouraged to reach maximum capacity and a posture improvement is the result. One word of warning here: for a warm-up to an activity other than exercise or as a means of taking a break, the stretches do not need to be held for more than eight seconds.

Group members stand against a wall. Are their shoulders flat? What position are the neck and head in? Where are the bottom and the heels in relation to the rest of the body? Partner work is useful here, with exploration and understanding enhanced by conversation and movement. Allow feedback from the partners to the group as a whole. Discuss what they consider is good and bad posture and allow them to demonstrate. Let everyone try until an agreed posture is arrived at from the group as a whole, they can then be shown the correct way of maintaining this posture through practice. Practice is the key: an agreed homework chore could be to practise this position, holding it for one minute each day. (Group involvement in decision making shortens the road to acceptance of good practice that is then maintained.) You could also have clients lying on the floor — particularly useful where someone has difficulty flattening the back.

Individuals walk across the room (if you are in a gym use the lines on the floor) with partners or the group watching how the body moves (and any bad posture) and focusing on how the person felt as they walked. People inevitably look down. To correct this you can place a small bean bag on their heads (first ascertain whether they have any neck problems, as weight can cause damage to the vertebrae) or get them to focus on something on the wall. With certain groups you could explore using a blindfold, but you need to be sure first of all that this does not cause anxiety. The blindfold encourages them to *feel* their bodily movements in a good upright posture. Only allow them to take seven or eight steps. This often makes them aware for the first time that some parts of the body do not appear to be in alignment.

Sitting in chairs, explore comfort and discomfort, enacting positions that family members or friends use. Holding them for a while and discuss them. Then choose one that feels good, demonstrate it to the group. Everyone takes a turn. The trainer then details the facts about alignment of the body, bones, muscles and so on, and explains why sitting in certain positions causes tension. The trainer explains effective ways of establishing the best sitting position, for individuals to practise on their own. The aim is to provide recognition of ways to relieve tension when working or trying to relax and a good body position that will enhance this.

Within a workshop, allow time for clients to stretch their bodies out in order to take a break and feel restored, stretching their arms above their heads, breathing in as they do so, lowering their arms as they breathe out. This can be done from a stationary position or while walking around the room. It encourages recognition of the productive effect that stretching can have on the body and of the individual's control of this physical reaction.

Observation of members of your group will highlight for you their bodily messages and posture. This knowledge will enhance your capacity to provide them with constructive self-help mechanisms that encourage relaxation and control. See if there are persistent body attitudes that they habitually assume when demonstrating some form of stress. Encourage them to acknowledge this; explore how they feel and whether they were aware of what they were doing. Encourage group participation and examine ways to change that can lighten the load of their stress. Whenever a member appears uncomfortable, use a constructive break, with breathing, stretching and walking, to restore their energy and capacity to continue. Comfort is the key to retaining our members.

Voice

The tone, volume, pitch and quality of a voice can establish or deter a cordial atmosphere at a first meeting with someone. The voice-box itself is able to project a large number of sounds, from high pitch to low, and to demonstrate clearly a full range of emotions.

A developmental aspect of understanding body messages is exploration of the role the voice plays in supporting or detracting from the intended message. The tone, volume, pitch and quality reflect our feelings and express our tension. We judge and are judged by others according to the voice tone that is being used. Indeed, we are more likely to respond to the tone of a voice than to the content of its message.

The advantages of relaxing the voice can easily be understood by clients when you have established with them where tension is felt when they are talking. In this way you can help them to recognize that relaxing the neck, throat and chest helps them to breathe more deeply and project their voice more fully with the least effort.

Teaching and learning aids

Exploration of the many different ways we use and interpret voices in everyday situations will help your participants to clarify and understand when tension is present.

As teachers and trainers you need to be aware of your own voice — its actual sound, the raising and lowering of pitch and the speed of your delivery. Tape-record yourself at home reciting a story, depicting a drama and trying to help an individual relax. Play the tape back, noting down what emotions are being expressed and how. Use this process as an appraisal system of constructive self-criticism.

Within a workshop format you can explore your own and your group's ideas of what constitutes a relaxing voice. For example, some people like a soft, slow tone, while others prefer deeper tones and a quicker pace. As a trainer you need to be flexible, developing a delivery that is both comfortable for you and responsive to your participants' needs. Watch them; ask them how they feel after relaxing; establish whether there have been any problems. By observing and evaluating the body messages of your participants you will be able, by adapting the sound of your voice, to improve your skills of delivery that will determine the success achieved through relaxation.

It is not necessary to speak all the time you are relaxing your participants. Pauses are an effective way of reminding individuals that they are engaged in relaxing themselves.

Words

Linked to the use of body language, body alignment and posture and voice tone is our use of words as a means of communication which may or may not help a person to feel relaxed. We are all aware of words that are cutting and meant to hurt as well as words that are loving and encourage confidence. Interpretation of these words is very subjective and may depend on the way they are said and the accompanying body messages. (Conversely words may be used to emphasize acknowledgement of body language.)

Let us start with the word 'Relaxation': in general terms it means feeling good. In workshops, individuals have used the words, 'firm', 'stiff', 'rigid', 'tight', 'tense', 'knotted', and 'heavy' to describe being unrelaxed and the words 'soft', 'loose', 'melting', 'light', 'flexible', 'pliable', 'calm', 'floaty' and 'tranquil' to describe being relaxed.

They notice tension occurs when they are tired, angry, afraid, pressured, depressed, feeling rejected, undervalued or feeling out of control in a situation. Tension is mainly experienced in the head, neck, shoulders, wrists, fingers and back, occasionally in the chest, stomach and toes.

They notice relaxation occurs mostly when they use a relaxation technique (occurring more often with more frequent practice), when they are happy, when they are being cuddled, when they feel loved, when they feel in control of a situation, when they like themselves and when they like others. It is felt all over the body and within the mind.

Often it is the delivery (tone) of the words that tempers their meaning, for example, 'I love you' said calmly, softly and with feeling may enhance a feeling of security, calmness, reassurance or desire. The same words, said loudly, angrily or with emphasis, can denote fear of rejection or a desperate need to be believed.

Teaching and learning aids

Self-development skills

Listen to the words, and the delivery of those words, of family members, friends or colleagues, reflect on the way you interpret them and ask whether your interpretation was correct. Keep these words and their meaning in a book. You will soon realize that the same word can have very different meanings and this will help you not to prejudge the meaning of participants' words during one of your workshops.

Start to recognize your own particular way of using words in order to get a point across, to clarify, challenge, impart information or to encourage openness within your workshops. This understanding will enhance your delivery, improve your use of words, increase self-confidence and add to your stock of knowledge and professional skills.

Workshop skills

I use words to heighten relaxation *after* I have dealt with participants' understanding of body language, body alignment and posture and voice tone. By this time participants are beginning to perceive aspects of change that they can control themselves and are becoming willing to explore other avenues to increase that control. For example, a relaxation format could include the use of the following sentences:

I am relaxing   I am peaceful   My mind is quiet

I am calm   I feel my energy restored   I am renewed

The key words could then be used on their own:

Relax   Peace   Quiet   Calm   Restored   Renewed

There are many ways of achieving, understanding and developing the use of words to make us feel calmer and more in control. For example, encourage each individual in a workshop to use one word to describe how they are feeling at that particular moment. Write the words down for all to see. Choose one of these words and ask each member of the group to say it. Encourage the other members to say how they felt the word was said: the tone, delivery and the body message. Explore other meanings of the word, seeking clarification as to the change that occurs when someone thinks of a different meaning. Finally, explore how participants felt physically, recognizing tension and relaxation within the word and its emotional delivery. The framework of the workshop becomes a foundation upon which to build participants' understanding of their personal use of words: what they are portraying when they use them; whether this is the message they wish to put across; and how they may misinterpret others' use of the language. This serves to reduce the tension that can be felt during conversations where messages are misunderstood, and results in a more relaxed approach to difficult situations.

A development from the use of single words is the use of whole sentences that encourage an individual to use positive realistic statements in order to enhance their relaxation. I usually use this technique at the end of a bodily relaxation session, with sentences such as 'I am letting the pressure out and the calmness in', 'I feel my body relaxing' and 'I am helping myself to feel good'. Autogenic training (see Appendix) also uses easy mental exercises designed to switch off stress and switch on relaxation. I use a form of this approach in my work because I believe the power of the mind activates our physical responses and therefore we can change these physical responses through practice of sentences that embody specific realistic beliefs, words that motivate us to relax. The main difference is that I do not tend to use repetition of sentences as a kind of mantra.

A development of the use of words and sentences is your ability to tell a story that encourages relaxation. Discuss first with the group what they like and any fears they have, and then use themes such as the seasons, the beach, woods, valleys, mountains, the weather, a trip to a favourite place, looking around the home, playing in the park, a fun fair or watching clowns.

Sense of smell

It is important to recognize that smell helps to determine our likes and dislikes. A smell may cause us to recoil in dislike, or move closer when pleased, as well as subdue or increase our sexual urges and behavioural mechanisms. Smell can therefore affect emotional behaviour.

Kristen Olsen, in *Alternative Health Care* (1991) talks of a research study at Warwick University which established the benefits of smell in inducing relaxation. Students in a laboratory experiment sniffed ozone and such coastline odours as seaweed and rotting clams in order that their responses could be tested. Relaxation responses in some students increased by up to 17 per cent.

Teaching and learning aids

Be aware of the facts that smells that are pleasant for some people may create allergies in others. Make sure you discuss allergies with your group before you embark on a workshop on smell. If you wish to develop your knowledge of effective aromas to aid relaxation you can learn about aromatherapy (see Appendix), or join one of the adult education courses which are run in this subject area. They tend to last for five sessions of two hours, although sometimes a one-day course is available.

Adults

I encourage my participants to bring in smells that they find relaxing. We then find out if anyone else likes them, what about them encourages or inhibits relaxation, whether a particular smell in a room is pleasant or irritating, and discuss any aromatherapy that the group may have used, such as perfume, bath oils, massage with oils or candles. A smell may be used during a relaxation technique to see if it enhances or hinders the relaxed state. The purpose is to acknowledge that we are all different, this difference being important to the level of relaxation that can be achieved by an individual. It may be that each group member chooses an oil that they like and tries it out in a bath, letting the group know in the following session how they felt. *Warn your participants to read labels carefully* in case of allergies or pregnancy.

In many situations with elderly people, particularly those who are confused, we can use their sense of smell to spark memories and encourage discussion, or indeed to reduce pain. Reminiscence therapy with elderly people aims to give them a sense of normality. Many elderly people become very tense and agitated when they are unable to remember something, and the use of smells may relax thought processes. Aromatherapy has also been used to help patients suffering from cancer to ease their discomfort and give them a sense of 'feeling good'.

Touch

Touch and massage have a relaxing effect on muscles by reducing stiffness, soothing nerves, toning skin and affecting deeper organs and tissue. We all use touch to demonstrate our feelings for others, but we also use acupressure on ourselves in many unconscious ways: reducing pain by rubbing or massaging; improving circulation to a particular limb; protecting ourselves from the sun by rubbing on oil. Massage can be used with all ages as a form of relaxation.

Touch is essential to our well-being and to our skills in interacting with others. Relationship problems in adults often stem from their lack of physical contact. I therefore stress the importance of contact with my clients.

Massage is generally not contra-indicated, but it is important that individuals are warned not to massage areas if they have large bruises, fever, inflammation, swelling or skin eruption.

Teaching and learning aids

Watch people: how often do they rub themselves; does rubbing soothe or hurt them? Try to be aware of your own body and the way you soothe it. Write down the different ways people massage themselves, then try them on yourself. Do they help or not? This will give you a greater understanding of the needs of the body and the list you have made, added to the list of examples of body language (pages 13-14) will provide possible workshop themes.

Massage is something that I have had myself and most of the time it has been wonderfully uplifting, soothing and relaxing. Only once have I experienced discomfort, when I had a massage which was very rough, creating tension rather than reducing it. The message here is to try massage yourself with a professional, on the understanding that you do have the right to say if it is uncomfortable. (See Appendix for further details on massage.)

Gentle massage can be used with all age groups. Unfortunately, when we reach adulthood we sometimes ignore ways of reducing discomfort and providing relaxation which we learned as children. Within your workshops you can work on simple forms of massage, first with individuals, touching, rubbing and soothing different parts of their bodies, discussing sensations, any areas of discomfort and so on. When moving on to partner work, trust is essential and you need to make it clear that no sexual stimulation is to be attempted. **Jane Madder** in *Relax and Be Happy* (1987), gives some good examples of techniques to use with children or teenagers.

You can also use the massage concept within your relaxation component. When the group is relaxed, use words that stimulate an image of participants massaging themselves or their partner, or of a professional doing this. Encourage their belief in its restoring, calming effect as the warmth of the massage permeates their bodies, enhancing their relaxed state. As I have said before, it is essential that you discuss the process you will be using with them before-hand so that any negative memories that may have prevented an individual from being able to relax in this way are reduced. If someone does not wish to participate, let them sit out and watch. They will have reasons for not wishing to take part that they may feel unable at that time to share with others.

I have used a form of massage as a stimulant in a warm-up for a dance session, with individuals rubbing all of the body in order to raise the temperature of the muscles, preparing them to work, providing comfort and stimulus to move. I have also employed a professional, who showed my group how to use simple massage techniques on each other. This particular group was made up of couples and it was agreed by them that they would like to know how to massage each other, particularly at times of stress. In this instance women were told to bring bikini tops and the men took their shirts off. This may cause problems for some individuals, in which case they can watch or try being the masseur. It was a very useful session as it provided the opportunity for individuals and couples to be aware of the control they can have in relaxing themselves and their partners. Self-esteem was increased.

Breathing techniques

Although breathing is the first and last thing we do in our lives, many people do not use their lungs efficiently. This is particularly true during stressful situations, where the tendency is to breathe shallowly. Learning and understanding the important part that breathing techniques can play as a means of coping during any stressful time will help your clients or group members to feel less tense and more *in control* of the situation. It will also be beneficial for you to practise these techniques yourself, so that you have a clear understanding of how they may work before you use them within your workshops. Often the individuals or couples I work with say they like the breathing best because it is the easiest, the quickest to show effect and they can do it at any time.

Some physiological facts

► The chest is full of muscles which pull the ribs up and down and enable us to breathe.
► We breathe in order to take in fresh oxygen, passed through our lungs, into the blood stream (pumped by the heart) and to the muscles that are required to work.
► Our lungs actually fill our breast cavity and should be fully used.
► Breathing is automatic, because it is controlled, like all our other internal functions, by the nervous system. However, it can be consciously controlled through special breathing exercises, which will override the nervous system. Because of this, breathing can be an effective tool in controlling some of our autonomic functions.
► The more oxygen the brain receives the more effectively it can function.
► Diaphragmatic breathing (explained in detail later) has three important effects on the body:

(a)   it fills the lungs completely, providing the body with sufficient oxygen;

(b)   it forces carbon dioxide, the waste product of respiration, out of the lungs;

(c)   the up and down motion of the diaphragm gently massages the abdominal organs, increasing the circulation of these organs and so making them function more efficiently.

► A relaxed state is characterized by breathing that is slow, deep and regular.

Some of the problems that individuals may encounter

A useful way of developing group involvement is to establish with participants whether they recognize the following signals in themselves or in others.

► Breathing rapidly and often, using only the upper part of the chest (may denote anxiety).

► Sighing frequently (may be a sign of depression).

► Anxious people tend to talk at the peak of inhalation, whilst depressed people talk at the end of exhalation.

► Tension, headaches, rapid heart beats (palpitations), sweating, dizziness or fainting (may be caused by stress).

► Shallow breathing, which does not use the lungs to their full capacity; if the demand for fresh oxygen is not sufficient to meet our body's needs this can lead to muscle fatigue.

► Body pain perpetuates fear, causes us to breathe shallowly and creates tension.

► Anger can make breathing irregular; fear and stress can produce quick, shallow breaths.

Contra-indications

It is important as trainers that you are aware of the contra-indications of breathing exercises. The most frequent problem is over- or under-breathing creating a sensation of dizziness. In the majority of situations this is due to a person not expelling the air sufficiently before the next breath is taken. Encourage your clients to exhale and inhale, fully and slowly. It is also important that you check if any clients are asthmatics or have a lung disease. Some asthmatics find deep breathing difficult, others do not. *A gradual process* of increasing the depth of the breath until a peak of comfort is reached will help the individual to become aware of any problems. If these are continuous, participants should refer back to their own doctor. I also find that individuals who have panic attacks, where they feel they cannot breathe properly, usually respond quite quickly, after the physiological facts of panic attacks have been discussed, to controlled breathing linked to positive realistic thoughts. This is best done on an individual basis rather than in groupwork, as panic attacks can frighten others. In all cases I encourage individuals to practise the breathing technique while sitting as a group, so that I can quickly ascertain any problems they may have. Possible answers to problems include the following:

1   Encourage your clients or participants *always* to consult their doctor if they have any breathing difficulties, even if they believe they are due to stress or injury. Talking about their symptoms, fears and anxieties with a professional will help them to alleviate the problem.
2   Help them to recognize that learning to use their lungs efficiently by practising breathing techniques, will enable them to:

(a)   reduce the workload of the heart and its need for increased oxygen, important during stressful situations;
(b)   release stress and relax the body (for example, taking a few seconds to breathe slowly, deeply and regularly may produce a state of relaxation);
(c)   promote stamina, providing energy when they need it most;
(d)   sleep better at night by promoting relaxation;
(e)   increase the capacity of the muscles to work harder and longer;
(f)   develop a general feeling of well-being;
(g)   short-circuit the stress response and promote relaxation.

Teaching and learning aids

What are these breathing techniques and when should we use them? Either tape-record these instructions or ask someone to read them to you. Choose a comfortable position in a chair, on a bed or on the floor with a cushion under your head and shoulders. Breathe in through the nose (fill your chest cavity — you will feel your rib cage rise up towards your shoulders). Breathe out through the mouth slowly (shoulders will drop down and relax). Repeat several times.

Although the above technique may have felt as if you were

breathing deeply, the next technique, known as 'diaphragmatic breathing', is much deeper and particularly useful when an individual has had a shock or feels depressed, extremely nervous or anxious. In order to understand the difference between the two techniques, put one hand on your chest just above the breast and one on your diaphragm just under the rib cage. Breathe normally and, as you do so, note which hand is moving. For the majority of people it will be the top hand. Diaphragramatic breathing is achieved when the lower hand rises as you breathe in and falls as you breathe out.

To try this, place one hand just above your waist, under your rib cage. Take a deep breath through the nose. (Try to make your hand push out with your muscles; if this is difficult, place your hand on your belly and try again.) Breathe out through the mouth slowly. (Allow the hand to sink down and try to push your lower back into the back of the chair, floor or bed.) Repeat several times.

You should now be able to feel the difference between the shallow and deep breathing. If you wish you can add to the diaphragmatic breathing a counting routine which will eventually enable you to breathe more deeply. For example, as you breathe in count to three and as you breathe out count to three. (It is very important to make sure that you do not hold your breath in order to count to three. Each action should take the whole of the three seconds. If you find this is uncomfortable, start by counting to two.) A further development is consciously to make a noise as you breathe out. The expelling of air in this way encourages you to take a deep breath in afterwards. Continue with these exercises two or three times a day and the benefits will soon be felt. If you experience a sensation of dizziness while breathing deeply you are over-breathing. Just relax and try to feel the chest expand to a comfortable level as it fills up and then expel the air immediately. It takes time to be able to breathe deeply and comfortably, but when you can the benefits are great. Your participants may find it helpful to imagine a balloon, filling up in the stomach as they breathe in and emptying as they breathe out.

In order to encourage group participation and learning I start with the facts about breathing, linked with constant practice so that, once they learn the benefits of using all their lung capacity and the good feeling it instils in them, they will start to do so automatically, especially when stressed. This constant practice can be continued throughout the workshop, just by reminding someone who is about to speak to the group, and who appears anxious, to take a breath before they do.

It is your responsibility to make each individual aware of the possibility of over-breathing. This can actually be a good learning phase for an individual. I have found that, where over-breathing has occurred, and they are able to ascertain the difference that correct breathing makes, they then use breathing very effectively in their lives. They actually feel more in control because they have recognized that they can change something that felt wrong within them.

The simplicity of this technique, which is just an enhancement of a natural everyday process, means that it can be used anywhere at any time. This needs to be emphasized with your group, using everyday examples. I may encourage group members to close their eyes and picture themselves in the situation that was difficult, feeling the emotions, then seeing themselves consciously breathing to feel calmer, noting any change to the image and the way they now felt. I encourage them to use the technique within a situation at work or at home which they recognize causes them problems and to tell the group how it worked at the next session. The feedback is always positive: the technique has worked or they had difficulty with it, which leads to a further practice and re-evaluation of the way they were practising it.

Where to use breathing techniques

In the car: every time we become anxious, annoyed, frustrated or tired, deep breathing will help to release the stress. If you are the driver and you feel a lot of tension in the shoulders, relax the hands on the steering wheel. Take a deep breath and, as you breathe in, raise your shoulders up towards your ears; as you breathe out, circle them backwards and let them drop down. Allow the back to nestle against the seat.

▶ *While walking:* correct breathing encourages a leisurely pace and promotes a general feeling of well-being, providing much-needed oxygen to the working muscles. It is best to use normal breathing while walking, with occasional deep breaths on stopping to admire the view.

▶ *While exercising:* correct breathing provides oxygen to working muscles and improves stamina and strength. *Never hold your breath when doing exercises, as this causes fatigue and can lead to injury.*

▶ *In bed:* breathing techniques encourage the body to relax, clear the mind and prepare the body for sleep. Some people find that, if they concentrate on the rising and lowering of the chest as they lie in bed (not the heart beating) it sends them to sleep. I use this a lot with people who have difficulty sleeping; most find it very effective and calming.

► *While practising relaxation techniques* (see next section): correct breathing releases stress, relaxes the body and promotes a general feeling of calmness and well-being. Calming thoughts will also help. For example, 'As I breathe in I let peace and tranquillity enter my body; as I breathe out I feel all my troubles leaving me.'

► *Before, during and after a stressful situation*: if you are in the middle of something and the phone starts ringing, take a deep breath before answering it. You will find you are much calmer and able to sound receptive to the caller. I use this particularly where work stresses are apparent. Participants who have tried this have said how it made them feel they were in control.

Also during an argument, when tensions are high, it can relieve the situation if each person takes several deep breaths before they reply to a comment aimed at them. They will find that they feel more in control of their words and even that the impact of any anger is lessened. Where illness is an issue and treatment is necessary, deep breathing techniques will enable an individual to feel more in control, relax the body and make the treatment process more comfortable and bearable.

► *When asking questions*: the desire to have answers is a very necessary part of our make-up, so it is natural that sometimes this desire creates anxiety about how to ask the question and get the full answer. Often this anxiety stops us asking the question at all or reduces its importance or clarity. By taking a deep breath before we speak, we gain a breathing space to think and provide the means to control our nervousness so that we ask the question that we really want answered. In these situations I also work on body language — how to sit, the use of eyes and so on — and on the selection of questions to ask.

► *When eating*: deep breathing encourages us to slow down our eating process, providing the digestive system with time to deal with each mouthful before the next one is swallowed. I have used this idea of digestion to enhance a relaxed state before food is consumed, so that food is seen as a source of enjoyment, relaxing and restoring energy and so that the desire to eat large meals is dissipated.

Relaxation techniques

As was seen in Section 1, there are many factors which can ensure that the ultimate understanding of how to relax is achieved. In order to reach this understanding it is important to establish *where, how* and *when* tension is present in the body before we look at the importance of releasing that tension, so that individuals or couples can understand and be able to feel the change when they achieve a relaxed state.

It is crucial when working with a client or group to be able to demonstrate the power of relaxation in creating self-worth and self-control. I therefore use lots of different techniques with individuals to find one that they feel gives them back a feeling of 'normality'. All of these techniques are initially based on understanding and releasing physical tension, with the optimum goal to create a sense of controlling the body and mind, to feel 'good' and able to cope. As practice is the key to good delivery, I often practise my own ideas. Trying different techniques yourself will enable you to experience the different ways that relaxation can be achieved.

I suggest that you discuss the facts of relaxation, as detailed earlier, with your clients *before* you show them any techniques, as I believe that theory aids practice and outcomes.

Contra-indications

Relaxation is a natural process that anyone can use at any time. However there are certain forms of relaxation that could cause problems to susceptible individuals. Be aware that some images which for the majority of people promote a sense of calmness will, for a susceptible few, create anxiety as a fear is rekindled. Take care with people who suffer from asthma or anxiety attacks or who have a smoker's cough, as they could have problems with deep breathing-enhanced relaxation. You need to encourage these individuals to use normal breathing patterns that gradually increase in depth as they become more aware of their bodies.

Tension-release relaxation is contraindicated for individuals who have heart conditions, or who suffer from high blood pressure or hypertension. These individuals should not tense any group of muscles for more than three seconds. However, in my 18 years' experience of working with these individuals, there has been a clear demonstration of the benefits relaxation can bring to their lives.

It has also been suggested that relaxation techniques may cause internal bleeding and acidity for some individuals who have gastrointestinal tract disorders, such as peptic ulcer or ulcerative colitis (see **Palmer & Dryden**, 1995).

Teaching and learning aids

It is most important to recognize that relaxation is personal to individuals, so be aware that some techniques will not work for you or your participants. The outcome of any technique will vary according to the individual's mood, when or where it takes place and for what duration of time. The important point is to try out the techniques and choose one that suits you. Try each technique at least three times before trying another one.

Basic (core) relaxation technique

Practise this technique yourself and use it as a basis for establishing the difference between tension and relaxation, as well as identifying where this tension is located in your body, thereby enhancing its effectiveness. There are two stages. Stage 1 serves as an initial format, stage 2 as a continuous format for the future. Note that there are two alternatives, with participants sitting or lying. Tape-record yourself delivering both, and then try them both out on yourself. Remember that voice tone and speed are crucial to the delivery of relaxation. This will be an ideal way for you to practise ways of voice delivery that will enhance relaxation. One constructive way of doing this is to count to three after reading each instruction to relax each individual part of the body. For example: *As you breathe in, press your feet hard into the floor. As you breathe out, relax them.* Now count to three as you breathe in and again as you breathe out. Then continue with the instructions.

When you play back the tape to yourself you will soon feel whether the speed and tone are relaxing you or if you need to speed up, slow down, increase or decrease the time between instructions.

Body alignment

Sit in a chair or lie down in a warm, quiet room with the light off or dimmed.

Sitting in a chair	Lying down
Sit upright, with the small of your back against the back of the chair	Lie on a bed, carpet or mat
Hands on your lap or the arms of the chair	Body in a straight position, head in alignment
Close your eyes to avoid distraction	Remove glasses if worn Close your eyes
Feet flat on the floor, slightly apart. Ankles, heels directly under knees	Have a cushion under your head/neck (and small of the back if you need it)
Take two deep breaths	Take two deep breaths *If you have a bad back, bend your knees and place your feet flat on the floor*

Listen to the noises outside and inside the room; let them drift over you, before and during the relaxation.

Start by tensing an area and then relaxing it, so that you can feel the difference between tension and relaxation. Once you understand this difference there is no need in future to create tension in order to relax yourself. This is *very important* when working with individuals or groups, as I have found that, if they continue to create tension in order to release it, they actually have a tendency not to release it properly, so tension is retained and the benefits of relaxation are hindered. However I use this technique first so that their awareness of tension and relaxation is heightened, explaining that this is an initial stage.

You may find it beneficial to repeat each exercise twice: try it, see how it feels; if it seems too long re-record yourself saying the instructions only once. If you or your students have not tried deep breathing before, it is very important to make clear the importance of *comfortable breathing*. Initially the majority of your participants will need to take more than one breath between instructions. It is only after considerable practice that one breath in and out can be taken for the full length of one instruction. Tensing of any muscle group is only held for three seconds (maximum).

In the following text the dots mean that you can prolong the

Stage 1: feeling the difference between tension and release

	Sitting in a chair	**Lying down**
Feet	*As you breathe in* Press your feet hard into the floor *As you breathe out* Relax … them	*As you breathe in* Flex your toes by pointing them away from you *As you breathe out* Relax … them and allow to drop to one side
Calves	*As you breathe in* Lift feet up until they are only balanced on heels, feeling tension in the calves *As you breathe out* Lower feet to the floor	*As you breathe in* Push your heels away from you *As you breathe out* Release heels and let feet drop to one side
Thighs	*As you breathe in* Squeeze knees and thighs together *As you breathe out* Relax … knees and allow thighs to separate The whole of the lower part of the body should now be relaxed and soft	*As you breathe in* Squeeze knees and thighs together *As you breathe out* Relax … knees and allow thighs to separate The whole of the lower part of the body should now be relaxed and soft
Buttocks/ belly	*As you breathe in* Squeeze buttocks together, pull your belly in *As you breathe out* Allow the buttocks to part and the belly to sink … into back of chair	*As you breathe in* Squeeze buttocks together, pull your belly in *As you breathe out* Allow the buttocks to part and the belly to sink … into the floor

Hands/arms	**Sitting or lying**
	As you breathe in Clench your hands into a fist and press your arms into your sides *As you breathe out* Release ... the fingers and turn the palms up, resting on legs (sitting) arms slightly away from the body (lying)
Shoulders	*As you breathe in* Lift both shoulders up towards your ears *As you breathe out* Allow them to sink down ... and away ... from the neck
Neck	*As you breathe in* Turn your head to your left *As you breathe out* Return to centre Repeat to the right
Face	*As you breathe in* Clench your teeth, screw eyes up tightly *As you breathe out* Unclench ... your teeth, lower ... the jaw, let the mouth open ... slightly and relax ... the eyes

preceding word by slowing down and emphasizing its meaning. Breathe normally now (not deeply) and feel relaxed in the whole of your body. Try to visualize in your mind your favourite place, somewhere where you always feel relaxed: in the bath, walking in the fields, listening to music in the sitting room, and so on. Picture yourself there and wallow in the wonderful feeling of contentment and the warmth that enters your body and relaxes it even more.

Coming out of relaxation
It is essential that you are aware of the need to come out of relaxation

gradually, as to do so quickly can create a greater sense of tension and put the person off trying again. Add this next set of instructions to your tape; as before the dots mean that you may extend the length of the preceding word.

When you feel ready to come out of the relaxation, do so in the following way.

Sitting in a chair
Wriggle your toes and fingers; lift your heels up and down. Rub your hands together until you feel the warmth in your palms; place the palms gently over the eyes. Open your eyes; feel ... the warmth; remove your hands and look around you. Stretch ... your fingers and circle your shoulders; take a breath; rise slowly to your feet; wait a moment. Have a good stretch ... raising your arms above your head (just for a moment). Walk around.

Lying down
Wiggle your toes and fingers.
Rub your hands together until you feel the warmth in your palms; place the palms gently over the eyes. Open your eyes; feel ... the warmth; remove your hands and look around you. Bring your knees up towards or over your belly. Take your right (or left) arm and bring it across the body, rolling from the hips onto your side at the same time. Use a whole body movement — no twist at the waist. Wait a moment; allow the blood to circulate; breathe ... Slowly ... up to a sitting position; wait a moment, breathe ... Up to standing, walk around and have a stretch.

If at any time during your relaxation you are disturbed and need to deal with a situation quickly, rise slowly and reflect on the fact that your calm feeling will help you to focus and deal with it. This is a very important aspect to draw to the attention of your group, as getting up quickly requires increased blood flow and is often the reason for a person feeling dizzy when they do so.

Stage 2: breathing-enhanced relaxation
Following on from the relaxation technique you have just practised is a breathing-enhanced relaxation for everyday use. Practising relaxation every day will provide the greatest benefit and ensure that we automatically draw upon it when it is needed at a stressful or

tense time. I suggest to my group members that they aim to practise the following technique at least every other day and, where possible, every day.

It is best with this technique to be lying down, but if that is really uncomfortable for individuals in your group allow them to start by sitting in a chair. Even when I have had individuals with back problems we have been able to find a way that they can lie down and feel comfortable. Initially you may find that some individuals do not like lying down because they feel out of control: you can soon spot this, as they tend to fidget and continually open their eyes. Simple discussion with them about these feelings, explored with the group, highlights the feeling of loss of control, which can be re-established by allowing them to sit and watch others, before practising in a chair or moving back onto the floor.

The following is the *main technique* that I use to relax my group members. As you read these words you will begin to see where emphasis on the tone of the word highlights and encourages relaxation: 'Experiment, see which words you feel enhance relaxation for you; try them out; change any that you are not comfortable with.' I do not stick to these exact words every time because often in group discussion you will be struck by a word or phrase members use in order to feel in control and transpose that into the relaxation session. For example, one group member described relaxation as a feeling of melting away like an ice cube, from cold to warm, other members liked this so I incorporated the words 'melting', 'cold' and 'warm' into my relaxation instructions.

The body positions are as they were for the previous technique, and as before the dots mean you can prolong the words if you wish to. Remind participants to use breathing patterns that feel comfortable for them. Developing the ability to take one breath in and out as the sentence is given takes time and practice.

Feet	Take a breath and as you *breathe … out* let your feet drop … away from you. They may feel heavy at first and then become lighter … and lighter … and lighter …
Calves	Take a breath and as you *breathe out* feel … your calf muscles sink into the floor. They may feel heavy at first and then become soft … and light …

Knees/thighs	As you *breathe in* this time turn your knees and your thighs out to the side and as you *breathe out* let them sink ... down into the floor. Take another breath and let them sink lower ... and lower ..., becoming lighter ... and lighter ... and lighter ...
Belly	Take a breath and as you *breathe out* feel ... your belly muscles soften ... and stretch, sinking ... down into the floor. Take another breath and as you *breathe out* feel them sink lower ... and lower ... any tension melting ... away, so that the lower back is resting comfortably on the floor.
Shoulders	As you *breathe in* raise your right shoulder up towards your ear; as you *breathe out* let your shoulder drop ... down and away ... from the neck, moving the arm away from the side of the body and turning your palm up to the ceiling, feeling the shoulder drop ... down even ... more. Repeat with the left shoulder.
Head/face	Gentle breathing now. Move your eyebrows up ... and away ... from the eyes; as you do so you will feel the skin around the eyes soften ... and relax ... with your lashes barely ... touching your cheeks. Feel your forehead relax ... and any furrowed lines drift ... back into your scalp. Then as if someone was gently ... massaging ... you, feel ... the skin across your cheeks and down the side of your jaw soften ... and become smooth ..., letting the jaw drop gently down towards the chest, the lips parting slightly as the teeth and tongue nestle ... gently in the mouth.

The whole body should now feel relaxed, with comfortable normal breathing. Focus on being in a warm, welcoming place that makes you feel good. See yourself there; feel the warmth and enjoyment entering your body.

Teaching and learning aids

Feedback is crucial to the development of your own personal skills as a trainer. There needs to be enough time at the end of a session for a quick review of how individuals felt before, during and after the relaxation, particularly any aspects they felt hindered their progression into a relaxed state. Evaluation sheets that include an opportunity to express their like or dislike of the technique will provide you with constructive criticisms and reinforcements of your practice, and enhance your abilities.

When I am working with individuals or group members I establish with them where their favourite place is, what it is like and how they feel when they are there, encouraging descriptions of the environment and the positive, calming effect it has on them. This then helps them to focus on the scene when relaxing and eventually enhances the length of time that they can maintain the relaxed state.

Once the body is relaxed, we can begin to focus on allowing the mind to relax. Participants can achieve this in various ways, using the aids detailed below. One word of caution: make sure that you stress the importance of your group members' not trying to think of things that would be frightening to them or would reinforce bad memories. For example, if you decide to set a scene such as a beach, it is possible that someone in the group will be afraid of water and become very agitated as the session continues. *It is imperative* that you establish any fears people have and be sure that you do not use them in a relaxation session. Many people will say that it is important to face fear in order to deal with it, but relaxation is meant to enable us to feel good, not bad. Dealing with fears is far more effectively handled within a discussion session of the group, when everyone can feel safe.

Listed below are some examples of imagery you can use with individuals or groups. Each of these should only last for a few minutes, particularly with a new group, as if they go on too long tension can return. Be sure to remind participants to breathe normally, not deeply, during the imagery phase. More detailed information on this technique will be found in the section on 'Creative imagery'.

▶ Imagine seeing oxygen as tiny bubbles, soft, floating clouds or a warm soft breeze. As you take a deep breath, feel the energy enter the body and as you breathe out see this energy in the form of bubbles, soft, floating clouds or a warm, soft breeze, passing down through the body, out through the feet, ready to be breathed in again. By repeating this several times, you will begin to feel more and more relaxed.

- Imagine going on a journey to a favourite place or somewhere you have always wanted to visit. Look around you; visualize everything there; enjoy yourself.
- Imagine you are on a bed of soft feathers that are taking all your weight. Feel the soft, floating sensation of secure weight-lessness.
- Think of an object, such as a piece of furniture or china, then visualize and feel its texture.
- Visualize a piece of gold, silver or crystal. Watch it change shape and colour as the sun shines on it; feel the warmth of the rays as they are reflected onto you.
- Imagine drawing or painting a picture using any medium; step back and admire it.
- Imagine baking a cake or cooking a meal; lie back and wallow in the smell and taste.
- Imagine listening to your favourite piece of music; allow it to soothe and calm you (you can have this playing the whole time you are relaxing the body, but very low and preferably without singing as voices tend to raise and lower awareness, creating tension).
- Visualize your favourite flowers, emerging from a bud to a full bloom, feeling the strength inside you as they grow stronger and stronger.

Another important aspect to remember here is that relaxation and mental imagery can decrease fear, through an individual re-gaining self-control and belief systems that recognize the power of the mind to alter a physical and emotional state to one that releases stress and tension, thereby creating in them an ability to confront and alter any sense of hopelessness or helplessness.

Art therapy

Often used in workshops, art therapy can also be used with individuals in counselling. It provides the means for individuals to express pent-up emotions by drawing, painting, collage and sculpting, in a safe, trusting environment. One of the many benefits of this therapy is the ability the medium gives the individual to grow in awareness about themselves or their partner. This releases inner tensions of emotions and leads to calmness.

When teaching children the fundamentals of art techniques in my early teaching career, I was often aware of the quiet, introverted or emotional child whose communication skills would blossom through their pictures. Often this is a clue to their inner feelings and the way they express them can heighten your awareness of the level of these emotions and how to deal with them. We all recognize a child's first drawings and, indeed, often heap praise upon the child for their efforts. This instils in them a belief that self-expression can be rewarded and fun to do, yet as they get older a lot of people tend to think their pictures should be an exact copy of an actual object or scene, which hinders their expressiveness and narrows the opportunities for new understanding to emerge.

Using art as a medium for expression in groupwork adds another dimension to an individual's exploration of the issues that are affecting their lives. It enables them to look at their beliefs from another perspective; it also invariably opens up a door to communication that for some might otherwise have been firmly closed.

Teaching and learning aids

The best possible way of understanding the vast possibilities of art therapy is to try it yourself. You can do this by joining a workshop or adult education class, or by reading books (see the Bibliography) and practising the ideas in them. When I was a group member of an art therapy course it was enlightening to be on the 'other' side. The experience was very rewarding both personally and as a technique to be practised within my workshops.

When using art therapy with individuals it is very important to provide the opportunity for them to explain what their picture means to other members of the group. In this way openness about personal feelings is explored and group empathy can be enhanced. Once an individual recognizes that this expression in both art and speech is a means of communication they will feel able, as they progress through life, to use such therapy again.

With individuals whose introduction to art was based on copying, trying to work in an expressive way that is free-flowing and not meant to resemble any particular object or scene can initially be extremely inhibiting. It is essential, therefore, to discuss first of all what the aims of using this medium are, by providing examples of your own or other people's work. Make sure you have their permission, especially if their name is on the picture, and ensure that the messages relayed from the picture are the ones that were voiced by the person, and not your own. In my experience the ones who are against this approach initially are the ones who benefit from it the most.

There is no need to think that your whole workshop always needs to be focused on art therapy: it may be that you use it within a session as a means of exploration. For example, if you were working on a relaxation technique and someone was having difficulty relaxing you could encourage the whole group to draw what relaxation and tension means to them. Allow each person to describe what their picture is saying or, if you are using partner work, ask the partner to describe what they believe the picture is saying, before the 'artist' says what it meant for them. The development is to establish whether anyone felt tense during the relaxation and, if so, how they could change this, so that they could achieve the relaxation they have depicted in their drawing. This openness enables a 'reflective' understanding of a person's beliefs and positive ways to challenge and change these beliefs, enabling them to feel in control and able to relax.

There are also advantages for an individual within a one-to-one session to have the opportunity to draw and explore their feelings. This is particularly useful where an individual has reached a 'block' in their understanding of what is happening and why, or is having difficulty explaining what they feel. Art therapy becomes a 'descriptive' process of enablement, yet another means of realising inner emotions that are heightening tension or stresses for an individual.

It is not necessary to have vast amounts of material. You can start with crayons and paper and then encourage individuals in your group to bring their own mediums to use. There are also lots of manmade or natural mediums that can be used at very low cost to make up collages.

Creative imagery

We already have natural skills to picture something that we are thinking about doing, such as having a bath. The enhancement of these skills of imagery is seen as a way of nourishing the mind by using these techniques as effective motivational tools for understanding ourselves: a self-enabler for people to use whenever we feel we want to reinforce or change a perspective or behaviour in our lives. (Practitioners use both 'imagery' and 'visualization' with reference to the creation of mental images. For the sake of simplicity, the word 'imagery' will be used in this manual. Readers who would like to know more are referred to the Bibliography.)

Children use imagery all the time. Within their minds there develops a capacity to see images of past or present objects or things which are useful stimuli for play development and comforters. Sometimes children see themselves as someone famous or as childhood heroes. This practice continues into adulthood and, as already seen, these imagery techniques have been used to enhance the relaxation process and encourage a developmental self-control in an individual's approach to life. However it is important to recognize that individuals have different abilities: some think in images, some sense things and others feel or think in words. It is practice that will enable them to develop their other abilities as well.

Contra-indications

The content of imagery exercises needs to be explored with the individuals before they are practised, in order to establish any fears or medical conditions they may have. For example, there may be severely depressed individuals who can only focus on the negative, individuals with a fear of water, or individuals who are injury- or blood-phobic and may faint. As long as you describe and explore the scene you will be setting, and receive feedback from the group about its comfort and safety aspects, they will be able to use the theme effectively.

Teaching and learning aids

In order for you to 'feel' the uses of the above techniques you need to practise them yourself. Begin by relaxing yourself (using a tape-recording, as suggested previously), a family member, friend or group member, using breathing and release of muscle tensions techniques, as imagery works more effectively when you are relaxed. If an individual remains tense then their capacity to deal with a negative image will be impaired, as the tension within their body implies that they are unable to change. The relaxation can be simple, especially if the person is in a chair. Some people start by relaxing the head and work down to the feet, but I prefer to go from the feet to the head as the brain is the last part that is being asked to relax and alter its perception to induce a calm state. Here is an example for you to use. As usual the dots mean you can prolong the word in order to induce a deeper relaxed state.

> Sit upright, with your feet flat on the floor, your back against the chair, hands resting on your lap and your head tipped slightly forward. [This should not hinder breathing; ask about any neck problems; comfort is the key.] Use conscious, comfortable breathing: as you breathe out allow a different part of the body to relax and as it does so feel the wasted energy (tension) being released into the atmosphere, out of the room.

Starting with the feet [as you the trainer say the following words, participants will be consciously thinking of breathing new energy in and pushing wasted energy out through the part of the body you are mentioning]: feel the feet soften and sink down, feeling lighter and lighter ... and softer and softer ...
the knees, calves, ankles, sinking down, softening, relaxing, more and more ...
thighs, buttocks, separate, sink ... down and relax ...
shoulders drop down, lower and lower ... elbows, wrists, fingers, soften ... and relax
eyes soften, jaw relaxes ... teeth and tongue nestle gently in the mouth.
Take five deep breaths (as deeply and as comfortably as you can without dizziness). As you breathe in, feel the fresh oxygen enter your whole body and as you breathe out feel the last bits of the old wasted energy released. As the energy flow increases with each breath, feel every part of your body growing stronger and more and more ... relaxed ... Tell yourself you feel good, ready and able to look at the image that you wish to cope with.

Once the relaxation is established you can use imagery as a reinforcement of a person's ability to cope with a certain situation that is causing them anxiety (also known as rehearsal). By imagining a stressful situation, they can confront it without panicking or retreating from the scene. These issues can just as easily be addressed in a group as in a one-to-one session. In fact in many ways working in a group enables a wider range of understanding to occur and builds bonds between group members.

It is crucial for you as a trainer to recognize that for imagery to be effective there needs to be discussion before and after the practice. You need to understand the issues from the person's point of view and they need to be able to believe in the possible changes that can occur. For example, when I teach breathing techniques I sometimes encourage a client or group members to focus on a particular time when they felt tightness or shortness of breath due to anxiety, reminding them of a time they have spoken about. They will often begin to feel the sensations occurring, but using the breathing techniques we will have practised they begin to see that they can diminish the feeling in their chest and in their image. This has proved particularly effective with individuals who have panic attacks, as it highlights the power of their brain to create physical anxiety and calmness within the comfort of a

45

session. Discussion afterwards highlights their recognition of their ability to alter their feelings into a more relaxed state, but also to open up the avenue for discussion on what thoughts were going through their minds at the time and how they changed when the symptoms began to subside. This enactment enables them to see that it was their thoughts that were causing the anxiety attack and by changing their thoughts to more realistic ones, linked with breathing techniques, they were able to change their physical symptoms and the attack subsided. Often this is quite a revelation for them and leads to a lot of opening up about emotions and thoughts.

You will find the use of role-play helpful with groups. An individual is asked to picture in their mind the way a particular person (one that they dislike) behaves and then to try to portray this themselves in a role-play with a partner. Discussion takes place as the partner relays the messages received from the role-play. This often enhances an individual's understanding and interpretation of the other person's behaviour and encourages them to look at their own behaviour and make changes that will help to ensure a calmer atmosphere is achieved whenever they next meet this particular person. This is very much linked to body language and would be a useful area to explore within a workshop centred around body language.

Dance

Being able to act out scenes, even dramatic ones, through personal movement allows the individual to release their innermost feelings. Expression, contraction and release enable an individual to be as one with their body. The diversity of moods of movement enables us to demonstrate and understand changes in our emotions.

All forms of dance are a relaxant: bodily movement increases adrenaline and blood flow and improves energy, strengthening and stretching muscles, improving posture and muscle control, all of which is conducive to relaxation. Using basic rhythms on a regular basis frees the body from tension and rigidity, releasing feelings, enabling a person to dance through their emotions instead of being stuck in them.

Dance is a medium for all ages that is fun and makes us feel good in our minds and bodies.

Teaching and learning aids

Reflect on what dancing means for you. Have you had good and bad experiences? Was it age, attitude, type of dance or the group you were with that made the difference? Write down your answers: they will help you to recognize qualities or difficulties others may have.

If you are new to the use of dance as a stimulus for relaxation, join a class or go to the theatre and watch as many different forms as you can: ballet, contemporary, jazz, musical drama. While you are there look around you, see the faces of those watching, what are the messages they are giving. Adult education in particular often offers a wide range of opportunities for learning new styles of dance.

For some of those in your workshops who seem overweight or withdrawn, dance may provide an initial or complementary form of communication. Many practitioners use the whole session for dance, with a quiet relaxation period at the end. For other practitioners who use dance as a form of relaxation within the main theme of the workshop, the dance element may last five to ten minutes, depending on the wishes of the group.

Linking mediums of expression together can often enhance the delivery of the main theme of your session. For example, if your session involves a lot of sitting and talking, providing breaks involving movement will provide stimulus for discussion. You can also dance as a warm-up technique or as a way of releasing pent-up emotions before a relaxation technique that ends a session. When exploring body language and posture, dance offers the opportunity to be expressive.

When choosing music, start with instrumentals, as singing can hinder natural expression. Use a wide variety of music. Some dance teachers use music as the main stimulus, others use it as the supporting element to a particular theme. It can also be interesting to have your participants bring their own music and spend five minutes on free movement interpretation of each piece.

Dramatherapy is a specialism on its own (see Appendix), but it can also be used to enhance dance movement as it provides an opportunity for adults to see in a different light situations which previously have engendered physical feelings of tightness and tension, and emotional feelings of anxiety and anger. Being able to portray feelings while acting as someone else is a comforting way of releasing these feelings and their connected tensions.

Music

Most people listen to music every day. It provides comfort,

relaxation and pleasure. It is often also used as a stimulus for those with disabilities, as it provides instant encouragement to move, and as an aid to reminiscence in encouraging elderly people to remember past experiences.

I have used music not only as a basis of support for my dance themes, but also as a means of enhancing a relaxed state.

Teaching and learning aids

Read about music and its applications for therapy. There are many good books related to remedial therapy for certain disabilities, and these give an idea of the possibilities of music.

Build up a library of music for all age groups, including instruments, vocals and those with a story basis. You could start with records from your local library, which will usually have a good selection for all age groups, and this will give you the opportunity to try them out before you actually spend money for them. Purchase tapes that are conducive to relaxation (see Appendix), or look around your book stores, which often have a selection of books on music at reasonable prices.

Use music as a stimulus for enhancement of a relaxation aspect of your workshop. For example, you can get your participants to sit or lie down and just listen to the music, focusing on the sounds entering the body and encouraging relaxation, or you can relax them first and then encourage them to listen to the music, allowing it to take them on a journey of pleasure. (Check first that the theme of your music does not have unpleasant associations for any of your participants.) Another possibility is to set the scene yourself and talk through a journey, emphasizing aspects of the music that enhance your scene. (Check with the group to ensure that they have no difficulties with such a journey.)

Be aware. Watch the group's body language. If there appears to be discomfort, *slowly* lower the level of the music until it drifts away, then discuss what it was like, any problems and so on. You could encourage group members to bring their own favourite piece of music, but you need to stress the importance of bringing music that does not have too strong a beat. This hinders relaxation as such music constantly changes rhythm and stimulates, even sometimes irritates, rather than relaxing.

Exercise

The word 'exercise' conjures up thoughts of physical movement, not relaxation, but it is through the stimulus of activity that a true resting state can be achieved, we recognize and feel the difference between tension and relaxation through exercise; we become more able to 'communicate' with our muscles, asking them to become supple and relaxed.

There is substantial evidence to show that exercise enhances the body's physiological state as it uses up excessive adrenaline created by stress. Indeed studies have shown that exercise is better at relaxing and elevating one's mood, without side-effects, than some widely prescribed tranquillizer. Studies also provide evidence to support the theory that vigorous exercise tends to stimulate the immune system, and helps us to see our body as a source of pleasure, something deserving of our care and attention.

The physical and emotional benefits of exercise

There is substantial medical evidence to suggest that exercise makes a major contribution to health in a number of ways.

- ► Exercise increases the efficiency of the heart.
- ► It strengthens muscles, joints and even bones, keeping joints supple and aiding mobility as we get older.
- ► It improves digestion and regulates our appetite.
- ► It promotes a good, erect posture and generates vitality and confidence, encouraging a relaxed state of body and mind.
- ► It lessens the problems associated with rheumatism, arthritis, diabetes, backache and depression.
- ► It reduces cholesterol: exercise is known to speed up the metabolism so that the body uses up more calories.
- ► Exercise and relaxation are felt by many people to give a tremendous feeling of well-being, relieving tension and stress.
- ► Regular moderate exercise will promote circulation and is believed actually to help lower blood pressure.
- ► Exercise makes us more alert, improves concentration and helps us to relax and sleep better. Sleepless nights are often associated with stress and tension. Exercise promotes a feeling of well-being and relaxation within the body, helping us to relax further, until we fall asleep. (However it is best not to exercise just before retiring, as this acts as a stimulant.)
- ► It is good fun and a way of making new friends and enjoying our leisure time.
- ► It gets easier the more we do it.
- ► It restores confidence in our own abilities, which in turn rekindles feelings of self-worth, demonstrating to us that we can

achieve something and have a role in life that can make us feel healthier, particularly at times when life seems difficult to cope with.

▶ Exercise speeds up the metabolism so that the body uses up more calories, and depresses the appetite, so that the desire to eat is curbed for a while. Exercise therefore is effective in reducing the amount of weight gain. You need to be aware that initially (especially if participants are very unfit) muscles will gain weight as they get stronger. Thus a person may appear to have lost very little weight, but their shape will be changing, their clothes will be looser, and they will feel better.

Teaching and learning aids

Practise yourself, 'listen' to your body and write down how you feel. How long does this feeling last? Does it suppress your appetite? Can you work for longer afterwards? Do you have renewed energy or do you feel exhausted? If you do feel exhausted, unable to do anything for some time after your exercise, you have done too much and probably with an exercise or activity that is not suitable for your needs. You probably do not like it much either.

A good exercise trainer has the ability to understand the different abilities and confidence levels of individuals and to ensure that whatever exercise is used can easily be broken down into stages that stimulate successful outcomes and encourage further participation. You will notice the person who does not participate well: they are often seen not to try as they fear ridicule. You can help them by ensuring that every task has a simplified element that provides instant success; this also encourages discussion that recognizes the importance of an individual's need to feel good about themselves, rather than competing with others. This recognition enables them to try harder, breeds confidence and provides the basis for understanding their bodies that makes them receptive to the introduction of relaxation as an enhancement of their ability to promote their own well-being.

Discuss with your group how they felt before and after an activity. This will enable them to focus on their physical reaction to an exercise and provide the impetus to watch for, feel and change physical tensions during relaxation.

Workshop ideas

Exercise can be used for most of a session, with relaxation at the end, or as a process of warming up or taking time out during a session. This applies to all age groups. For many teenagers, exercise is a confidence booster that begins a process of feeling good. Competitive and non-competitive elements will encourage recognition of the benefits of personal fitness, as well as the sharing, caring, working with others approach that is paramount to a good workshop. In most instances this age group like most of the session to be taken up by exercise, with a component for relaxation at the end, but it is important for them to be able to recognize in other groups the benefits of exercise as a form of break that induces a more relaxed, attentive state.

With adults you need to be aware that they may bring to the sessions ingrained theories and practice. The most withdrawn will often resist attempts to get them to exercise. This is the time to use the evidence of the benefits of exercise to encourage discussion, followed by simple exercises in order to warm up at the beginning of a session or to act as stimulants for concentration throughout a session. Always explain what the purpose of each exercise is and discuss participants' thoughts afterwards. I believe this provides a basis for understanding and self-control, expressed as 'If I want to feel better, exercise will help me.'

Every session should comprise a warm-up, a main theme and a cooling down. The importance of this is to provide a safe basis of exercise that will not cause injury. I also make a point, after an exercise session, of introducing relaxation, which I see as a way of continuing the cooling down while enhancing the participants' feeling good. Every group I have ever worked with has said that the relaxation part of the session is like 'being rewarded for having worked hard', a chance to reflect on what they have achieved.

Explore the general benefits of exercise with your group members, as detailed earlier, but be aware of specific needs. For example, if participants have a general feeling of stiffness, using simple exercises that will reduce this stiffness will provide an avenue for change that they can continue to use outside the workshop.

Understanding the barriers
People will bring with them to a workshop many stereotyped arguments that reinforce their belief that exercise is not important. Discussing challenging and clarifying these arguments will not only encourage your participants to exercise but will instill in them a confidence in your ability to help them to help themselves. The following are some of the comments they may use and ways you can challenge them.

▶ *'I am already very active rushing around'* This rushing around really constitutes pressure, sometimes very stressful, causing the body to feel tired, the mind to be overloaded and the outcomes not always as we would wish them to be.

▶ *'I don't have the time'* By not allowing time for ourselves we lay ourselves open to feeling tense, agitated, and often of little value: continually striving to put others before ourselves leads to emotional and physical fatigue.

▶ *'I don't enjoy getting sweaty'* Sweating is an essential process in promoting our well-being. Besides, emotions, thoughts and feelings make us sweat and feel uncomfortable as well as exercise.

▶ *'I don't like competing'* There are many non-competitive sports, where the only competition is with ourselves to get fitter and more skilled.

▶ *'I'm a warm weather person'* Exercise raises the body temperature; it is inactivity that makes us feel the cold!

▶ *'I'm too old for it!'* Age makes no difference. The benefits of exercise are felt by all; good circulation is particularly important as we grow older.

▶ *'I don't need it'* Are you really listening to your body? How hard was it to get up this morning? Does your back ache quite often? Do you get tired more easily?

What exercise to choose

It is important that participants like what they are doing. If a particular exercise becomes a chore, it is time to think about a different one, but encourage them to make three or four attempts at an activity before they decide it is not for them.

Dos and don'ts of exercise

▶ It is important to wear the appropriate clothing for the activity. Use a good pair of shoes that feel comfortable and give support, especially around the ankles, and lightweight outfits that keep the person warm without creating too much heat. Trousers of any kind need an elasticated waist, otherwise they will restrict movement. Jewellery should not be worn.

▶ Warming up allows us to prepare the joints for work, improves the circulatory system by raising the body temperature and blood flow to the working muscles, and prepares nerve and muscle response patterns, thus preventing muscular soreness and injury. A warm-up should include *gentle* movements as well as deep breathing techniques.

► Over-exertion will cause fatigue and, possibly, injury. This is particularly so for people who have not exercised for a while. Some people find competition invigorating which is fine as long as they can accept that they may lose. The dangers of wanting to win at all costs are self-evident. Those who feel physically unwell should avoid exercising until their body has had time to get rid of the germs; but if feeling unwell is associated with feeling depressed, participants will find that exercise will lift them.

► It is important not to hold your breath while exercising. In sit-ups, for example, I teach individuals to breathe in when the body is open and breathe out when it is constricted. Holding the breath is often associated with pain, and some believe that working through pain is the best way to get fit. *Pain is a warning to stop what you are doing as it is likely to cause injury.* It can also be a sign that you have not warmed up properly. A good exercise session should make us feel good, not exhausted or unable to walk. There is no truth in the belief that only exercise that leaves us feeling sore the next day is worthwhile.

► Do not exercise within an hour of eating.

► Use a few stretching techniques within exercise-based routines. They enhance the individual's ability to develop their own physical skills and at the same time allow for reflection (others may call this meditation) on restoring energy and feeling good. This can be particularly useful at the end of a session where you feel your group need some time to reflect about the session and how they feel.

Stress management

All my workshops, whatever their theme, include relaxation and stress management techniques. They may be used initially to encourage participation or to reduce an identified stress that a person has shared with the group. Relaxation techniques have an important role to play in reduction of pressure and stress management techniques have a strong role to play in removing barriers that may hinder relaxation.

Herbert Benson, in his book *The Relaxation Response* (1976), asserts that 'profound relaxation turns off the chronic release of stress chemicals from the brain so the body can focus on normal self-healing'. It has also been recognized that stress is a consequence of constant arousal and muscular tension, unconsciously learned and often habitual, dictated by our unconscious beliefs about who we are, who we should be, the way others are and the way the world should be. Stress has been defined by physicists and engineers as 'physical pressure exerted upon or between parts of a body. Strain occurs when the equilibrium between the two parts is lost and strain or undue pressure is felt'.

Pressure is an important part of our everyday lives. It often provides the stimulus to creativity and can be a challenge, a spur to action. It is when the pressure turns to stress that we need to examine the effect it is having on us.

The aim of stress management workshops is to provide a means of looking in depth at the causes of pressure and stress in an individual's life, in particular stress that is felt to be unmanageable. The objective is for each individual to identify these stresses and to be helped by different techniques to recognize within themselves their own personal ways of coping and to add to these new skills that can be used in the future whenever the need arises.

Teaching and learning aids

There are many courses available which teach stress management techniques. There are also numerous books on this subject (see the Bibliography or your local library for suggestions).

Stress workshops (more than one session) should include the following:

► What is stress? What is stress management? What does stress mean to an individual?

► What are the physical, mental, emotional and behavioural symptoms of stress as identified by each individual?

► Which of these happen often, are difficult to deal with or are often avoided?

► Understanding and recognition by individuals of situations where they can and cannot cope.

► Finding personal stability zones and rituals; when and where they are used and what they could be used for in the future to reduce stress.

► Re-establishing individuals' personal, practical abilities to help them get through difficult situations.

► Learning new skills to reduce stress and feel in control.

► Within a group framework, the opportunity for individuals to share with others situations where they have recognized stress in themselves and to seek common ground and possible solutions.

The many different issues which will surface during a session will include success and failure, self-worth, negative thoughts, comments of others, avoidance, managing loss, time management, unrealistic goals, lack of communication and physical symptoms of stress.

One of the most important aspects of stress management is the ability of an individual to acknowledge the pressure to which they are subjected and its manageability, rather than avoiding it until it becomes severe. If a headache is beginning to be felt, ignoring it and hoping it will go away may merely make it worse, while taking a break, walking away and using breathing techniques will reduce its intensity, promote circulation and restore energy, so that the person is ready to continue.

Acceptance of personal limitations eases the pressure of needing to be seen to be successful, as well as recognizing the reality that learning is a continual process. It also provides the opportunity for a person to replace negative thoughts with positive ones. Unrealistic goals can be dealt with in a workshop. Establish that long-term goals that have no chance of realization tend to heighten, not reduce stress, while continuing to point out the importance of short-term, *achievable* goals which can provide immediate pleasure and the impetus to continue in a series of successful stages.

Dealing with failure is something that we have all had experience of at some time or another. What is important is not the failure but the way we feel about ourselves afterwards. Participants need to be shown and to accept that it is OK to fail. It is also crucial for them to reflect upon the fact that we can learn through failure. We frequently exaggerate the importance of failure. Instilling a sense of proportion is a way of diminishing in a participant's mind the 'awfulness' of a situation that is preventing them from being able to deal with it constructively.

Stress at work

Frequent breaks are an important means of restoring energy. All too often we work through any lunch or tea breaks, even when we are working at home. Within a workshop feelings of tiredness, fatigue, depression, fear of rejection or fear of failure may be heightened as the result of an individual's wrongly held belief that taking breaks is wasteful. We therefore need to demonstrate to participants the validity of taking breaks and their usefulness as a way of restoring energy and releasing tension, and as an acknowledgement of our personal needs.

Dealing with avoidance

Avoidance encourages a person to believe that they will feel more in control and less stressed if they avoid dealing with a situation. What really happens is that this avoidance leads to feelings being bottled up until they can no longer be contained and are released at a time that has little relevance and with a vehemence out of all proportion to the situation which set all this in train. This issue always surfaces in workshops, so you can use examples from group members to demonstrate the benefits of dealing with rather than avoiding a situation. The aim is for an individual to recognize that avoidance achieves nothing except more anguish, particularly if they are faced with the situation again when they cannot avoid it. Facing the situation will help them to focus on ways of coping and dealing with it, making it bearable, and will prove to them that they can stand it and diminish its effect.

Physical stress

Relaxation techniques can be used to address the problem of insomnia or to control sweating, which often accompanies anxiety.

Time management

Time management techniques enable participants to avoid the pressure to cram into a day as much as they can because they feel 'they should' and the anxiety and self-criticism that accompanies failure. These techniques include the following:

► learning to put themselves first, allowing time for themselves to recharge their batteries and increase their capabilities to finish their work: relaxation is very useful here as it provides the opportunity for personal time;

► ensuring that individuals are aware of the importance of time to socialize with others, time for working, time for relaxing, time for reflection;

► short-term, manageable goals: one of the key elements of successful time management is living for the moment, putting energy into what we have decided to do now and not worrying about future tasks for which we have set aside time;

► organizing time systematically.

Alternative therapies

We should never use a specialist skill that we have not been trained for, but that does not mean that we cannot look at the benefits they may provide for individuals. We should therefore provide access to information on all forms of alternative therapies, their purpose and practical implementation, written by professionals in the field, together with details of the main recognized professional bodies, to any individual who wants to know more about their uses. See the appendix for details of therapies, addresses, books and visual/audio aids.

When I set up a range of five-week courses offering introductions to alternative therapies such as Bach flower remedies, aromatherapy, reflexology, relaxation, homeopathy and stress management, the take-up was usually quite high. People are interested in learning new ways of reducing tension and relaxing, so if you are interested in any of these areas contact your local adult education centre to see what they are offering.

GUIDELINES FOR GOOD PRACTICE

Development of personal skills as a teacher or trainer of relaxation

A desire to learn about relaxation techniques and alternative ther-apies sends you on a journey of discovery, with knowledge acquired through joining courses, trying out the skills on yourself and supplementing this personal practice with theoretical understanding by reading books on your chosen technique. This process highlights the importance of continued learning, enhances clarity of thought and understanding, and develops specialized delivery skills.

There are various courses that offer skill-based training in relaxation, but usually within a stress management framework, as provided, for example, by the Centre for Stress Management, 156 Westcombe Hill, London SE3 7DH (Tel 0181-293 4114) or Pilgrim Training, 12 Park Road, Kempston, Bedford MK42 8NZ (01234 855316). In other cases relaxation is a component of another main theme, such as yoga. In these instances you need to contact the central body and find out more details (see Appendix). I have not yet found a course that centres solely on relaxation as a training base, but I am hoping to set up such a course with a qualification in the near future.

Aim to understand your own body, voice, mind and choice of words; where and when tension is present or absent. Use this ability to understand your participants' behaviour and emotions within a workshop to enhance your personal ability to alter moods that are not conducive to learning, concentration and sharing.

Strive to heighten your skills of observation, listening, diverting, facilitating, directing and demonstrating with constant practice and evaluation of your workshop, its specific aims, its broader objectives and outcomes, as well as your personal skills as a trainer. You can use your own thoughts, written down after a session, forms filled in by the participants or you can tape-record the whole session and listen to it afterwards.

Through learning in this way you will begin to be able to produce a 'portfolio' of particular needs of participants that high-lights physical and mental capabilities or disabilities, use of termin-ology, body language and behavioural tendencies of society in general and of individuals in particular, as identified when under stress. Acknowledge differences and find constructive ways to include techniques that will meet individual needs, such as those of a person with impaired hearing.

Practise breaking down your activities into stages that are

61

conducive to constructive, achievable learning, promoting confidence and a willingness to explore. Allow time for general as well as directive discussion.

Seek to establish recognition that no-one is or can be perfect, and that failure is never absolute. Encourage individuals to accept themselves as they are by exploring their beliefs about success and failure, perfectionism and the learning process.

Be clear about the content of the workshop and the possible outcomes obtainable by individuals.

Make sure that you have some quiet time for yourself to go over your notes, relax and regain energy, using positive thoughts and beliefs about your ability to deliver the coming session. Some people find it is very helpful to visualize the session and the way they intend it to run, as this often highlights problem areas, as well as revealing possibilities for the development of familiar ideas and the introduction of new ones.

Recognize your limitations and specialisms. Seek help or refer individuals on to other professionals where an issue needs to be dealt with in a session that is outside your skills base. If you are using another therapist, recognize that they will wish to be paid and who is to pay them.

Organizational abilities

Setting up the room

Be aware of health and safety requirements. It is your responsibility before every session to check any dangerous equipment, stacked chairs, slippery floors, stuck windows (open or closed), overhead obstructions, loose tiles and so on.

Ensure good ventilation, but beware of draughts. Relaxation is best achieved if a person feels warm. Use clothing or mats placed by the bottoms of doors and close windows (unless it is a very hot day) when practising relaxation.

Ambient temperature should be 60–70 degrees for a session to be comfortable. (When using exercise as a theme, it does not need to be above 50 degrees.) If the room is too hot or too cold, there may be loss of concentration and tiredness, and relaxation will be very difficult to achieve. If the room is warm enough for the main theme but not for the relaxation, allow your participants to put on an additional item of clothing or to cover themselves with a *light* blanket. Tell participants beforehand of any specific clothing they need to wear, such as trainers or tracksuits.

Blinds and curtains may be closed for privacy, but do not then turn out the lights for your relaxation session before you have discussed whether anyone has a fear of darkness. If you leave the lights on, encourage participants to close their eyes; otherwise they may feel blinded or uncomfortable. Rooms that have a dimmer switch are a great advantage, as you can adjust the amount of light to a level that is comfortable for the group.

Check that chairs and mats are available so that individuals can sit or lie down for the relaxation part of your workshop. If there are no mats available, encourage your participants to bring in their own. Yoga or lightweight exercise mats are the best. I also encourage them to bring in a pillow to put under their neck and shoulders as I find this helps them to feel comfortable and able to relax.

Try for a quiet room, away from constant sounds. If this is not possible, encourage your participants to disregard any sound by focusing their attention from it. Recognize the possibility of interruptions, as these will disturb your group. You can put a notice on the door saying 'Workshop in session, do not enter' or 'Relaxation in progress, please pass quietly'. Be aware of a room where the acoustics are poor: you will soon know if they are, as people will fidget. Check then to see if they can hear you. To overcome this problem you could use a microphone so that everyone can hear when they are lying down. You should also move around them quietly to ensure they can hear. Acoustics will also affect the quality of any music you play, so again a microphone will help: you can actually lower the sound.

Negotiate with the group to establish whether it is to be an open or closed workshop and to ensure that confidentiality will be maintained by the group.

Check any equipment you want to use, such as a tape-recorder, before the workshop begins and be prepared to use a back-up, to do without, or know where to get one.

Time management

The timing of the session will vary, depending on whether you intend to have a single introduction workshop, a continuous workshop or a short-term workshop. An introduction to relaxation workshop should last at least two or three hours. A one-day workshop where many different techniques are introduced could last as long as six hours. A continuous workshop — that is, a workshop occurring once a week for an indefinite period — should last one-and-a-half to two hours. A short-term workshop (lasting about five weeks) could be for two, or two-and-a-half hours a week.

Include breaks in your timing: one should be sufficient in a two-

or three-hour session. An all-day workshop should include two small breaks and a lunch period (of at least an hour). The shorter breaks can be for refreshments and for stretching the legs (no more than 15 minutes). Alternatively you could use a different activity to provide the break, such as an exercise routine to loosen up the body after sitting and before returning to sitting. Not every group wants a break when one is programmed. Whatever the circumstances, try to be flexible and provide the break at the right time for your group, which may not necessarily be the time allocated on your workshop plan. Remember that a break can last just a few moments (a few deep breaths with stretching and standing). The aim is for participants to appreciate the importance of a break as a restorer of energy and an aid to relaxation, whatever its duration.

You need to be aware of the different capabilities of your participants, their level of tension and their ages, and to bear in mind the session's duration and whether it involves sitting or standing, before you organize the type of relaxation you will be demon-strating. To achieve a clearer understanding of what is involved, show different ways of relaxing that take different lengths of time to complete, starting with a minute, moving on until an individual or group can practise relaxation for 15 minutes and then encouraging them to practise at home until they can relax for at least 30 minutes.

In a single session of three hours, aim to show them at least three different ways of relaxing within different time scales. In an all-day workshop of six hours you could show them at least six different ways of relaxing with different timescales. In a five-week workshop with a two-hour session each week, you could show them a wide variety of relaxing techniques, adding aspects that they would like to know about, taken from alternative therapies or from ideas of their own.

Work on the principle that group involvement is the key to good practice: make sure you allow time at the beginning and end of each session for the group to share their feelings. If it is the first session, ask what their expectations are before it begins and whether they have been met when it is over. In subsequent sessions, ask them to share experiences of using the relaxed techniques, to say whether these helped in the situation, how they are now feeling about them-selves and whether anything has changed. This sort of exchange often triggers other people's thoughts and makes them aware of changes of which they may not have been fully aware. It also enables us as trainers to establish where we may have given the wrong impression or not elaborated enough about something.

Encourage the use of warm-ups as they provide the comfort

zones (not only physical but mental) that provide the impetus for individuals to want to learn and take control of themselves. The timing of warm-ups depends on the main theme of the workshop, but they should last at least five minutes. Where the theme is exercise they should last at least 10 minutes. Cooling down time offers time for reflection. Always use a relaxation technique to achieve this, allowing between five and 15 minutes, depending on what you have been working on.

Aim to have sessions at the same time and day for the duration of your course. This enables individuals to plan and prioritize this time, which is important time *for them.* Timings are not set in stone, so do not feel obliged to stick to them. They are meant as guidelines to help you plan constructively, but they must also allow for creativity and flexibility. If sometimes a particular issue needs more or less time than you have allowed, this does not mean a failure on your part: it is more likely to be proof that the participants are involved and achieving something.

Presentation and delivery

Presentation

Produce leaflets that are concise, written in laypersons' language, give the required information and are easy to read. Using coloured paper is a good way to draw attention to a leaflet. Decide what the course is for, who it is aimed at and how you can reach them. Do you need external support, such as doctors' surgeries, clinics, newspapers, magazines, hospitals or social groups? Do you use an internal system of support, such as that of nurses on wards, to encourage patients recovering from illness to look at the possibility of joining a course on relaxation by giving them one of your leaflets? Do you visit yourself, talk to people and then leave them your leaflet? This can be very useful, particularly if you agree to give a one-hour (lunchtime) talk to a particular group of people on the benefits of relaxation. Make sure that the leaflet states what the course entails, who it is for, when and where it is to take place, for how long, at what time, any special clothing needed, directions to the venue and any cost. Coloured A3 paper (laminated as it lasts longer) is best for a notice board but coloured A5 paper is best for handouts.

Visual aids are a very useful tool to complement your workshops. They attract the attention of participants when they enter the room, and provide reassurance and evidence of your professional credo. You can make them yourself or purchase them from specialist organizations (laminate them so that they will last for years). Ensure that the information displayed is not only what you believe but what other professionals in that field believe. Overhead projectors are also useful, especially if you have a large group, or if they have sight or hearing difficulties. Have some large sheets of paper ready (old wallpaper will do, but not the ready-pasted sort as it can stimulate allergies) with felt-tip pens and Blu-tack or something similar to stick temporarily.

Have handouts ready to distribute at the end of the session, detailing the theory behind your practice. This provides an opportunity for your participants to check what has been said, to clarify and deepen their understanding of the theory, and encourages more practice. Also have a simple form ready that will enable each participant to evaluate the session and your practice. A sample evaluation form is provided at the end of this section.

Delivery

Position yourself where everyone can see you. Never have anyone sitting behind you, as they will only see your back and could misinterpret your signals. Best is a semi-circle or full circle where you can sit anywhere and mix in with the group. I favour *standing* when I am trying to impart theoretical information, using a projector or visual aids, or when writing the feelings of the group onto a large sheet of paper on the wall, and *sitting* when there is a general discussion or while showing a relaxation technique. Be prepared to be flexible. Watch your group. They will soon let you know if they are uncomfortable and if you need to be more directive — or, indeed, to negotiate what occurs next.

You will gain and hold the group's attention when you are able to present your information in a voice that encourages concentration and a desire to listen. The right pitch, depth and clarity are crucial to group involvement. Ask people if they can hear you. Encourage them to speak out if they need greater clarity. If people appear to be distracted, raise your voice, use humour, offer to reiterate what you have said, ask if there are any questions or points that you may not have explained properly. You can test this by asking a question about something you have just said, or simply asking if everyone understood your last point. Watch the body language: you will be able to see if there is a lot of discomfort. If so, try making the point again, but using different words. When rapport has been established, it enhances your sessions to have someone question you because it shows that they wish to understand more fully and it gives you a chance to practise your clarification skills! Actively encourage your group members to question you, pointing out that you learn from them as they learn from you. When standing to clarify information on a chart, do not talk consistently all the time you are looking at the chart, as your words may be lost: keep turning towards the group as you speak. Participants will learn through your demonstrations to review the way they speak and the words they use that have had a tendency to be misinterpreted by others.

There is no doubt that at some point you will hear individuals say something that is totally against your own beliefs. Sometimes this is done to test you, rather than because this person really believes what they are saying. Your body language and tone of voice are crucial here: if you demonstrate shock, disbelief or even dislike you will have lost the argument before it has begun and prevent others feeling that they can be open with their views. A relaxed atmosphere is enhanced where individuals can feel free to express their feelings and be able to accept any challenge that ensues. On very rare occasions a comment may be so destructive, particularly if it is aimed at another group member, that the person who has made the remark has to be asked to leave. It is often possible to ascertain from the person who has delivered the remark what lay behind it. Often it is a misinterpretation of another person's body language or tone of voice. Once this is established, the situation is quite quickly eased and better understanding is the result.

The pace at which you work will determine the natural progression of learning that can take place within a workshop. Remember that your projected time format for each aspect of the workshop is not immutable: it should be adapted to meet the responses of the group to any particular theme. This flexibility is very important as it enables your participants to feel a part of their own development and, in educational terms, it imparts a negotiated curriculum aspect in your workshop. Having said that, it is also important to ensure that the main theme of your workshop is explored, and this you can do by being directive. Thus a group that wishes to continue to discuss a certain topic can be given the choice of doing so for a set extended amount of time, or of returning to it if there is time at the end of the session, or of having it as a major topic in the next workshop.

Encourage discussion after the delivery of a major point so that clarification and understanding is achieved, using evidence of past experiences of both yourself and members of the group. Look at the components of your workshop: how much involvement of the group is there? Can you improve on this? The more participant involvement you have, the more individuals will feel able to open up and share their feelings. It may be that, initially, you favour a directive approach with a few practical interventions and then, as the group establishes itself, a more practical, discussion-based involvement. Or you may prefer to have group interaction immediately. Practice and evaluation will show which is right for you and your participants.

Ensure that your participants are aware of the importance of checking what the required qualifications of alternative therapists are with their professional body, before they consider making an appointment.

Be prepared to take on the role of a facilitator or indeed a group member. Both may be necessary, depending on your theme and the numbers in your group. Last but not least, be prepared to learn from your mistakes. This is the essence of a good trainer, someone who is able to reflect on their practice, listen to others' criticism without damning themselves and alter their practice accordingly.

Sample evaluation form

The following evaluation form is *an example* of the kind of questions I would ask of individuals in my groups. As this book is based on relaxation I have chosen to limit the questions to this theme. However in many of your workshops you will be using additional ideas to enhance a relaxed state and therefore you need to ensure that you ask questions related to that aspect. In most instances I try to keep the questions to one page and no more than 10–15 in number, keeping them simple without the need for long, analytical answers, as I feel this can cause stress for some people.

In order that I can learn from you about the suitability and structure of this course, I would like you to complete the questionnaire below.

Listed below are the main areas that were covered during our session. Please use a circle to indicate whether they were helpful or not on a scale of one to 10 — one not very helpful or detailed enough, 10 very helpful, or anywhere in between.

Do you have a clearer *understanding* of what tension actually is?

1   2   3   4   5   6   7   8   9   10

Have you been able to *identify* tension in yourself?

1   2   3   4   5   6   7   8   9   10

Where is it in your body?

Have you a clearer understanding of *body language* in relationship to the tension displayed by others?

1   2   3   4   5   6   7   8   9   10

Will you try out the *relaxation techniques* you have learnt on yourself?

Yes/No (delete where appropriate). State which ones

Did practising with a partner and watching their body language help you to understand the tension caused in others by the sound of the voice?

1   2   3   4   5   6   7   8   9   10

Was it a surprise to you to hear how your partner perceived tension in you?

Yes/No Please state why and if you agree with what they say

Can you see the important part the voice plays in creating or releasing tension?

1   2   3   4   5   6   7   8   9   10

Do you feel you will now be able to think about your own use of voice and body language in situations that you have previously found difficult?

Yes/No

Have you found it helpful to *practise* the relaxation?

1 2 3 4 5 6 7 8 9 10

Did the trainer's *voice* relax you?

Yes/No/Sometimes Does it change tone too much?   Is it too soft?
Too loud?   Do they talk too much?   Is it just right?

Have you a clearer understanding of the *breathing techniques* and their uses to help relieve stress and promote a feeling of being in control?

1 2 3 4 5 6 7 8 9 10

Do you think you will be able to use these when you feel stressed? Which ones in particular?

Do you think you will be able to include breathing in the rhythm of relaxing each part of the body?

1 2 3 4 5 6 7 8 9 10

Did the relaxation at the end of the session using the power of thought words help you to relax?

1 2 3 4 5 6 7 8 9 10

Has the approach of the *trainer* been of assistance to you?

Yes/No

Was the *delivery* of the session by the trainer:

boring? exciting? too slow? too fast? lacking in detail? too detailed?
interesting? excellent? just right? (you may circle more than one).

What grade would you give the session?

1 2 3 4 5 6 7 8 9 10

SECTION 4

PRACTICAL WORKSHOP IDEAS

Introduction

This section provides a wide variety of workshop activities to stimulate and add to your own ideas. They do not need to be followed to the letter, though you may find this useful to begin with. Experiment: try them out, change or disregard them, but keep practising. Practice is the key to effective, stimulating and successful groupwork. If you wish to explore this area further, the Bibliography lists suitable books. The section is in three parts.

Warm-up

Warm-up enables your participants and yourself to prepare mentally and physically for the session. It should prompt a sense of comfort, fun and relaxation. Each session should include an update and evaluation by the participants of the previous week's warm-up. Participants usually like repetition, so do not change the warm-ups too frequently: allow them to explore the benefits first. There are lots of different aids to stimulation, but I prefer not to use equipment for warm-ups, as I find that equipment slows down the whole process and is often better used as a support for the main theme.

Main theme

The first two workshops in this section centre around the main theme of relaxation. The remainder of the activities may be used with the main relaxation theme or are main themes in their own right that incorporate relaxation techniques to support their delivery. When you feel confident with your practice you can work at combining themes, according to the needs of your group. This creates greater stimulus and increases your ability to deal with different issues in one workshop. Throughout the main theme section you will see that, although the heading may be, for example, 'Stress Management', the activity may contain elements of other techniques, such as visualization, breathing or relaxation. There are many activities in which role-play is used, but it is not necessarily used in every workshop. The views of the group and the level of ease and empathy that has been achieved have to be taken into consideration. I do not use role-play for an initial session, as many people can feel intimidated by it.

Relax down

The relax down section is a simple way of endorsing the main theme by using relaxation techniques to enhance the state of being in control and feeling good. The duration of these activities depends on the group, the warmth of the room and whether or not this is a first session. As a guideline, aim to take between five and 15 minutes.

WARM-UP 1

Aim: Exploring the reality of tension as perceived by individuals
Age: Teenagers/adults
Time: 10–15 minutes
Equipment: Large sheets of paper with sentences written on
   them explaining what tension means and where it can be felt.
   For example, 'Tense means tight as a spring'; 'When I am
   angry my face is tense'; 'When someone is about to hit me, I
   go rigid'

■ Activity

1   As each individual enters they go over to the sheets and read
   them, before going to the centre of the room and sitting down.
2   Each person repeats one of the sentences and explains what it
   means to them.
3   One person demonstrates what the sentence means to them in
   a certain part of their body. Everyone else tries out this idea
   (usually very funny).
4   Simple relaxation techniques exploring the use of breathing to
   release tension (see 'Breathing techniques', pages 26–31).

WARM-UP 2

Aim: Enjoyment, recognition of the possibilities of using rhythm and body movements to warm up

Age: Teenagers/adults

Time: 10–15 minutes

■ Activity

1 Tap out a rhythm on your body to a beat of 1,2,3, 1,2,3, then 1 pause, 2 pause, 3 pause.

2 Choose different body parts to do the tapping on.

3 Join up with a partner. Tap out the beat on yourself; your partner copies the taps and the beats on the same body parts, either at the same time or in sequence.

4 Tap out the rhythm together, touching each other once through each beat cycle.

5 Join another pair. Synchronize the rhythms so that you all work at the same time, on yourselves.

6 Make up a simple routine using the rhythm where one follows the other until all four have completed the rhythm on themselves; then all four repeat the rhythm at the same time.

WARM-UP 3

Aim: Recognition of warmth and cold; empathy, understanding and caring (best used when group empathy has been established)

Age: Teenagers/adults

Time: 10 minutes

■ Activity

1 In a space, individuals rub themselves all over to create warmth.

2 Walking around, they meet a partner and rub each other's arms/legs/hands/backs.

3 Each pair, walking quickly, meet another pair; they huddle together to create warmth.

4 Each person in turn decides on one movement to keep warm and the others copy, intertwining, twisting and turning around each other to keep warm, huddling together.

WARM-UP 4

Aim: To heighten awareness of using energy, stretching and releasing to feel good and relaxed within a co-operation context

Age: Teenagers/adults

Time: 10–15 minutes

Equipment: Mats, hoops, benches (if available), bean-bags

■ Activity

1 Participants sit together and the theme is explained: the object is to get around the room and use every piece of apparatus before the whistle is blown.

2 Participants have to touch all four walls (mats are placed away from the wall so that they need to reach for it); step inside each hoop, bring it over the body and put it down; travel only on the mats – not touching the floor; place a bean-bag on their head and walk along the bench without it falling off.

3 In twos with one person leading, participants maintain contact (holding hands or coloured bands — these allow greater distance between the two) while negotiating the obstacles. Change over and repeat.

4 Discussion on what was difficult; how the body changed; what was needed for balance.

WARM-UP 5

Aim: To heighten awareness of good and bad posture
Age: Teenagers/adults
Time: 10–15 minutes
Equipment: Mirrors if available

■ Activity

1 On entering the room each person stands in a space, allowing shoulders to be limp, head lowered.

2 Taking a breath, they raise their head and shoulders, feeling taller. They repeat, this time stretching their arms above their heads.

3 Walking around, shoulders down, head lowered slightly, they simultaneously take a breath, lift their heads and shoulders, and stretch their arms above their heads, lowering them as they breathe out.

4 If mirrors are available, each time they a face a mirror they stretch up, breathing in, raising their shoulders and heads, looking at their body posture and alignment.

5 If there are no mirrors, they can either count to 10 as they walk and then breathe in and stretch or do so every time they meet someone face-to-face.

6 The group face inwards in a circle, moving together inwards, shoulders limp, heads down. As they reach the centre, they take a deep breath, lift shoulders and heads up, focus on the person opposite, look at their posture and smile.

WARM-UP 6

Aim: To provide comfort and empathy by learning about and introducing another person

Age: Adults

Time: 10–15 minutes

Equipment: A board, large sheets of paper, pens

■ Activity

1 As each person enters the room they read the message on the board, which tells them to sit down next to another member of the group and find out things about that person, writing them down if they wish to.

2 They establish who they are, what they do for a living, why they are there and what they hope to get out of the workshop. Each individual is to be prepared to talk about their partner.

3 The whole group is assembled and each person gives a brief description of the person next to them and what they are hoping to get out of the workshop.

4 Name labels are made and put on (first names only, large print, felt-tip is best).

5 The trainer gives a brief description of themselves, the aims and objectives of the workshop and makes a list of what each individual is hoping to get out of the course. This is displayed for the whole duration of the workshop and evaluated at the end.

WARM-UP 7

Aim: To establish our tendency to prejudge without evidence
Age: Adults
Time: 10–15 minutes
Equipment: Cards or sheets of paper, pens, name labels

■ Activity

1 Participants wear (first) name labels.
2 Everyone writes on a piece of paper or card what they would like to have done other than their chosen career.
3 Answers are placed in a hat in the centre of the circle. Each person picks out one (putting it back if it turns out to be their own).
4 In turn, participants try to guess whose alternative career they have picked out. (This is very enlightening and can be lots of fun.)
5 This continues until everyone is recognized and they have been able to say a few words about their desire.

WARM-UP 8

Aim: To encourage communication
Age: Adults
Time: 10–15 minutes
Equipment: A board, large sheet of paper, pen

■ Activity

1 On entering the room, each individual writes on the board what they hoped to get out of the session.

2 They put on first name labels and walk around the room, listening to a piece of music. Every time the music stops they are to ask the nearest person to them what they were hoping to get out of the session and explain what they are hoping to get from it. Repeat several times.

3 With the whole group sitting, discuss ideas people had when they first came in. Are they still the same or have they been altered or reinforced through discussion?

4 Review of the aims and objectives as perceived by the trainer and by the group members themselves.

WARM-UP 9

Aim: Opening up and awareness of body movements, good and bad posture, alignment; confidence building and empathy

Age: Teenagers/adults

Time: 10–15 minutes

Equipment: Bean-bags

■ Activity

1 On entering the room, take off your shoes. Walk around on your toes, then your heels, then heel, toe, heel, toe — not too fast. (The trainer to watch for cramps.)

2 Bend your knees as you walk on your toes, straighten your legs as you walk on your heels. (The trainer gives the sequence, such as four on the toes; four on the heels; four heel, toe.)

3 With a bean-bag on your head, walk with your body in alignment, shoulders back, arms by your sides. Smile when you meet someone.

4 Discussion of the body. What was conducive to smiling and what was not? How was tension felt? Where? When was it felt?

WARM-UP 10

Aim: To be able to seek out problems and share them in a workshop

Age: Teenagers/adults

Time: 5–10 minutes

■ Activity

1 The group sit in a circle relaxing, backs against their chairs, feet firmly on the floor, hands on laps, eyes closed, heads tipped slightly forward.

2 They breathe gently and then as deeply as is comfortable without feeling dizzy.

3 They focus on the oxygen entering the body, rejuvenating them, providing calmness and security, pushing out all the waste energy, or nervousness about working in a group. They think about recognizing their ability to be open and frank, with the desire to explore feelings with others, to learn together and change where desired.

4 They come out of the relaxation by slowly raising their shoulders, feeling good, calm, reassured, comfortable. They open their eyes, wiggling their toes and fingers.

5 Discussion of any aspects that were uncomfortable, any fears people have about working in a group.

WARM-UP 11

Aim: To use breathing and relaxation techniques to warm up and create group harmony before a session begins

Age: Teenagers/adults

Time: 10 minutes

■ Activity

1 The group sits in a circle, relaxing their bodies, by the use of breathing techniques focusing on energy entering the body and waste leaving it. (See pages 44–5.)

2 As the body begins to feel revitalized, each person reaches out to touch the hands of another. Gently holding hands, they feel the energy passing through their bodies, receiving energy through their left side and passing it on to the next person through their right side.

3 They allow the energy to fill the room, creating harmony and comfort.

RELAXATION 1

Aim: To enable an individual to acknowledge and understand the physical difference between tension and release of a particular part of the body

Age: Teenagers/adults

Time: 2 hours

Equipment: Mats, pillows (participants to bring their own)

■ Activity

1   Establish what participants' expectations of the workshop are; the trainer makes a list.

2   Exploration of the evidence about relaxation and tension (see pages 3–7) linked with 'Recognizing Tension'. The trainer makes a list of any identified areas of tension for participants at the present time.

3   Practice of a relaxation technique in a chair (see pages 35–6): tensing and releasing.

4   Feedback: exploration of feelings, differences felt, any areas of tension still felt. Make a list of situations where similar tensions have been felt by individuals. Discuss the benefits of the practice of tension and release.

5   Practice of relaxation in a lying position (see pages 35–6): tensing and releasing.

6   Feedback: evaluation from group, how they felt, differences between sitting and lying, which they prefer, any areas where tension still remains.

7   The trainer now gives participants final relaxation practice that encourages release from their natural state, rather than tensing first, so that they can practise at home. (See 'Relax Down 1'.)

RELAXATION 2

Aim: To establish the benefits of using breathing techniques to
enhance a relaxed state
Age: Teenagers/adults
Time: 2 hours
Equipment: Mats, pillows (participants to bring their own)

■ Activity

1 Reflection on the past week: how participants are feeling, any
changes, how often they have practised, any problems, and so
on. Use sitting relaxation exercise to release tension.
2 Exploration of facts about breathing (see pages 26–7).
3 Practice of normal and diaphragmatic breathing.
4 Relaxation in a chair using breathing technique instead of
tension and release (see pages 38–9).
5 Feedback: discussion from group. What are the benefits of the
two techniques; which feels easier and releases the most
tension?
6 Looking at situations where participants feel tense; anxieties that
they identified in the previous session; any new anxieties. The
benefits of using breathing relaxation in these situations.
7 The trainer explains that relaxation using breathing techniques
can be for one minute or longer. Practise techniques of one to
five minutes to calm the individual, restore energy or provide
the confidence to deal with a situation. For example, take five
deep fresh energy-giving breaths, pushing stale energy out
through the toes, at the same time allowing the body to soften
and relax; take two deep breaths, releasing the shoulders,
before answering the telephone; take one deep breath and say
to yourself, "Speak slowly and calmly" when faced with
aggravation from another person.
8 Evaluation of session, followed by relaxation using a breathing
technique: see 'Relax Down 2'.

BODY LANGUAGE 1

Aim: To recognize individual bodily traits, the ways messages are projected to others and how they can be controlled

Age: Teenagers/adults

Time: 90 minutes

Equipment: Chairs

■ Activity

1 The group sit on chairs in a circle. Each person in turn focuses on a person opposite them. Looking at the way they are sitting, each participant says what messages they feel are being given. (The person in question makes no comment.)

2 General discussion, starting with what the person who was giving the message actually meant or felt. Shared exploration of these meanings: who agrees, who does not, what the differences were. Reflection on ways we can misinterpret signals.

3 Look at everyday examples of body language that express anger, sadness, happiness, pride, anxiety, or which say: don't touch, cuddle me, I feel a fool. Each of these is portrayed by a member of the group. (The trainer may need to demonstrate first.)

4 Allow several people to enact the same message. Discuss the differences.

■ Development

1 Explore body language that could change the way individuals feel. The trainer needs to appreciate the difficulties of teenagers and the perceived misinterpretations of parents, teachers and peers.

2 Make a list of all the possible difficult situations individuals encounter and get them to show the body language they believe is used in those situations to the rest of the group. Allow time for discussion about the messages and any possible changes.

BODY LANGUAGE 2

Aim: To follow on from previous session to develop an understanding of body language

Age: Teenagers/adults

Time: 90 minutes

Equipment: Chairs and mats

■ Activity

1 With the group sitting in a circle, on chairs or mats, look at the evidence about body language: how we use it; what messages are given and received. Look at lists of examples of body language people use, establishing what participants or others use that is either comforting or welcoming.

2 Use group members' examples of good and bad body language, role–played by them. Here the trainer can show possible alternative interpretations of the message so that the group can discuss both.

3 Look at ways of changing these messages. With partners, participants practise changes to body attitude that promote comfort and self-confidence.

■ Development

1 Taking situations described by individuals, act them out in pairs, so that each person can try what they consider is the negative approach and then change it to a positive one.

2 Each couple demonstrates the different body messages and explains what they mean to them, before the whole group discusses them.

BODY LANGUAGE 3

Aim: Following on from previous sessions, to understand body language

Age: Teenagers/adults

Time: One and a half to two hours

■ Activity

1 Discussion of previous understanding of body language; group members discuss any that they have become more aware of since the previous session, using demonstrations where appropriate.

2 Explore with the group the feelings that are present in positive and negative body language, asking for demonstrations from individuals or explanations of how these feelings are interpreted by them.

3 Using examples of everyday occurrences to demonstrate body messages linked to emotions, let everyone act one out: shopping, breaking something, learning a new skill, and so on. After five minutes' practice, half the group demonstrate while the other half watch and vice versa. Discuss the messages received and the emotions that appeared to be present.

4 In pairs, participants role-play other examples: for example, courtship signals, welcome or rejection, meeting someone for the first time, being told off. Each individual chooses an emotion, such as anger, indifference, sadness, fear or happiness, and links it to the body language. Demonstration to the group is followed by discussion of the messages, both physical and emotional.

5 Look at ways of reducing the effects of these expressions with breathing techniques and changed thought processes. Group members try them out in pairs to see if they change their feelings. Outcomes are reported back to the whole group. This is followed by general discussion.

■ Development

Looking at ways of changing a negative message into one that may still be negative ('I'm not interested') but that is not seen as destructive by the person receiving it.

BODY LANGUAGE 4

Aim: Recognition of colours which reinforce our messages to ourselves and to others
Age: Teenagers/adults
Time: One and a half to two hours
Equipment: Scarves, hats, bags, umbrellas, clothing

■ Activity

1 Participants sit in a circle with lots of clothing, bags and so on in the middle. They have already been encouraged to wear their favourite outfits and to bring along a selection of others (with teenagers you may need to specify no underwear!) they like and do not like.

2 General discussion of favourite colours and how participants feel when they wear them (strong, in control, happy, vibrant, wild). They demonstrate how they move when they wear a particular colour. (At first, allow them to exaggerate as much as they like.)

3 Colours they dislike: participants discuss how they feel, and demonstrate how they move when they wear them.

4 They explore differences, choosing different colours, putting them on and seeing how they feel and how they move in them.

5 Partners discuss what messages each is receiving from the other's choice of clothes and colour.

6 Feedback from pairs is followed by discussion by the whole group on the way a colour can enhance or detract from the way we feel and the way we move. Participants look at the benefits of this exploration and the positive ways of using them to give the messages we want to relay.

RECOGNIZING TENSION 1

Aim: To understand how tension is created and to seek ways of changing it

Age: Teenagers/adults

Time: 45–90 minutes

Equipment: Various objects to hold: ball, sponge, bat, scarf, sandpaper, pen

■ Activity

1 In pairs, participants clasp and release objects, feeling the difference between light, firm and intense pressure. They watch each other, describing what they see: colour of fingers, hands, shoulders, jaw, general body language.

2 Group discussion of feedback from pairs on how they felt and what they saw.

3 Evidence of tension: its purpose, any positive or negative effects it may have on the body. (See pages 3–4.)

4 Recognition of individual cases where tension has a negative effect; examples are given by the trainer and the group. Practical ways of alleviating this tension are discussed, such as actively releasing fingers from a tight position, using the thumb to touch each finger in turn several times, rotating wrists (stimulates circulation), aiming for a lighter touch on picking up the object the next time. All practise this.

5 Participants use breathing techniques to clear their minds so that the different parts of the body relax and messages are more clearly received. Discussion of the use of this technique when an individual recognizes uncomfortable tension.

RECOGNIZING TENSION 2

Aim: To recognize that tension within the body during illness will prolong the recovery period, causing stress and anxiety

Age: Adults recovering from illness

Time: One to two hours

Equipment: Art materials, mats, pillows, chairs

■ Activity

1   Individuals are encouraged through listening to the facts about tension and the benefits of relaxation to explore where, when and how this tension is felt by them, recognizing in particular whether this tension was greater during their illness, the treatment itself or while waiting for the results of tests or operations.

2   Breathing and relaxation techniques are practised to lessen the impact of tension.

■ Development

1   Reflection and general discussion of the positive or negative results of practising breathing and relaxation techniques on their own.

2   Use imagery to enhance participants' relaxed state and encourage them to feel able to accept the treatment with realistic expectations.

3   Participants use paints or pencils to draw their idea of a 'saviour' (as they perceive the treatment) to take away their illness. They show their artwork and discuss it with the group.

4   After simple relaxation in a chair, they use the visualization of their picture to attack the bad cells, with the good cells devouring the bad, and feeling them melting away through the glands in the body.

RELEASING TENSION 1

Aim: To understand and accept the body's need to release emotions and the calming effect this has

Age: Teenagers/adults

Time: 60 to 90 minutes

Equipment: Pen and paper, chairs

■ Activity

1 Discuss different ways of showing emotion, such as crying, shouting, withdrawing, staring, glaring, smiling or laughing. Make a list of the ways in which the group recognize emotion.

2 Practise these emotions in role-play, allowing each person to choose two from the list made and enact them. Follow up with feedback to the group, demonstrations and discussion of feelings that are engendered by seeing other people's emotions.

3 Partners aim to show opposite emotions: if one cries, the other laughs; if one whispers, the other shouts; if one stares, the other looks away; and so on. They feed back and demonstrate to the group. This is followed by discussion of each emotion and the messages that were received.

4 Group discussion of the importance of releasing emotions and, thereby, tension, seeing positive ways of doing this that are not destructive to someone else or to themselves. Learning to deal with rather than avoid a situation.

5 With role-play, practise recognizing the release of emotion: when one partner releases emotion, the other actively aims to understand and defuse it by reacting in a different way. Feed back to whole group.

RELEASING TENSION 2

Aim: To appreciate, understand and use more actively the medium of laughter and singing

Age: Teenagers/adults

Time: 20 to 60 minutes, depending on age

Equipment: Mats and chairs, paper, pens

■ **Activity**

1 Establish what individuals find funny; make a list on a sheet of paper.

2 The trainer provides evidence of the benefits of laughter, adding the thoughts of the group: for example, it lights up the face, makes us look younger, draws people to us.

3 In pairs, participants discuss what makes them laugh or smile, even when they feel down. Coming back together, they all share these experiences.

4 Group discussion on ways to change our moods through laughter, such as watching cartoons or films, going out with friends, reflecting on past funny events, smiling or laughing at ourselves, challenging the thoughts that are creating anxiety.

5 Focus on the warmth of feeling that singing provides, or the use of relaxation and imagery of a time that they found funny.

6 The participants go away with several ideas to practise for altering a mood that they find creates tension.

VOICE 1

Aim: To recognize that voice tone, volume, pitch and quality all affect the way we are perceived and received by others, as well as belief in ourselves

Age: Teenagers/adults

Time: 60 to 90 minutes

■ Activity

1 Sitting in a circle, the group discusses the uses of the voice and people's interpretations (see pages 20–1).

2 Practice within the group, of voice tones and their meaning for the person speaking and for those listening. The trainer first gives examples and demonstrations. Then it is the group's turn.

3 Recognition of voices that are comfortable, irritating or threatening and ways of reacting to them. For example, with someone who shouts to gain attention, the reaction is either to ignore them, to shout or to speak more softly. Explore the outcomes of each.

4 By means of discussion and practice within the group, establish an effective 'voice' that enables an individual to give and receive messages without being tense.

5 Look at connections between body language and voice. In pairs, participants work on achieving body language and voice that create a feeling of being in control but in a calm manner, using examples from everyday occurrences.

6 Practice of a relaxation technique (sitting in chairs) for just five minutes, with the trainer using different voice tones to relax participants. Follow this by group discussion of which tones relaxed and which created tension.

7 As homework, ask participants to watch and listen to other people, noting down any particular use of voice tone, volume, pitch and quality that they have heard and which they can bring back to the group.

MAIN THEME

VOICE 2

Aim: To develop the previous theme of understanding the power of the voice to deliver messages by using this understanding to create awareness of the ability to relax by controlling the voice

Age: Adults

Time: One and a half to two hours

■ Activity

1 Reflecting on the previous session, is there anything the group has noticed others do with their voice that is different from or the same as what they do with their own?

2 Participants reflect on the body language connected with these voices and act them out in pairs. They then feed back to the group. Discussion of the messages received by group members.

3 Establish whether tension was present and discuss how it can be released: breathing technique, conscious lowering of the shoulders, facing the person when they speak, lowering or raising the voice, increasing or decreasing speed of delivery; and so on.

4 Participants look at situations in their lives where someone else's voice tone and body language have been difficult for them to deal with. They look at ways of changing this by challenging negative, unrealistic thoughts and changing their own body language and voice. Participants practise in pairs and then demonstrate and feed back to the group.

5 The trainer induces full relaxation, using tone of voice and speed of delivery to enhance the release of tension and promote a relaxed state. (See 'Relax Down 1'.)

VOICE 3

Aim: To understand the power of the voice and ways of using it that encourage a positive response from the listener

Age: Teenagers

Time: 20–60 minutes

■ Activity

1 Discuss the different ways we use our voices, such as whispering, screaming, giggling, shouting, laughing or crying.

2 Through practising these voices, ascertain whether tension or relaxation is felt in the neck, shoulders or body.

3 In pairs, participants role-play the vocalizations that are often rejected, such as shouting and screaming, and then those that are often well received and given attention, such as laughing, singing or talking calmly. One person in each pair chooses the negative, tension-creating one and the other the positive, relaxing one. They are enacted simultaneously, to see how it feels to have someone react differently to them, they then change over. The participants feed back to the whole group, with demonstrations.

4 Participants act out a drama with set words that encourage them to think about how they can say things in a calm, comfortable way that feels good and is receptive to others. You can use everyday activities, such as shopping or preparing a meal.

VOICE 4

Aim: To recognize the ability to calm and relax someone else
with one's voice
Age: Teenagers/adults
Time: 60 minutes

■ Activity

1   Following on from the previous workshop that explored an
individual's ability to create tension or relaxation, focusing on
using the voice to relax others.

2   In a circle, participants reflect on previous exploration of voice
uses linked to body language and how they feel about them.

3   The trainer demonstrates a simple chair relaxation technique
(five minutes).

4   Sitting in pairs, one participant listens to the voice of the other
as they try to relax them. Each person tries out two voices: one
they feel would irritate, and one they feel would relax their
partner (maximum five minutes). They then exchange roles.

5   Pairs feed back to the group: how each person felt, which voice
relaxed them (if any), what was missing. Group recognition is
established of a voice that promotes relaxation.

6   Participants look at situations in which they could use this voice
to comfort a friend, partner or family member, or to relax a
child. Examples are elicited from the group of situations in
which they have done so or in which they now realize it would
have been beneficial to do so.

7   For a relaxation technique (laying down), the trainer uses a
calm voice that prolongs the length of certain words in order to
enhance the relaxed state and so demonstrate the importance
of speed of delivery when creating relaxation.

WORDS 1

Aim: To isolate words we use to illustrate feelings and desires
Age: Teenagers/adults
Time: One to two hours

■ Activity

1 Sitting in a circle, discuss the use of words, their meanings and opposites, using a list provided by the trainer as a starting-point, supplemented by suggestions from the group.

2 Working in pairs, each person chooses five words, using each of them in a sentence that they believe makes clear their meaning. Their partner listens and then suggests possible meanings. They discuss.

3 Feedback to the group is followed by general discussion about words chosen and what had been found out about them.

4 The trainer establishes that body language and tone of voice play a part in the delivery of the word, its meaning and interpretation. (See 'Words' in Section 2.)

5 In pairs, participants act out a scene using body language and tone of voice to deliver their chosen word. They then feed back and demonstrate to the group. Follow up with a general discussion on the different messages that can be received from words, depending on the delivery.

■ Development

Look at instances where interpretations have caused anxiety to the person who is speaking or receiving the message. Are they the correct ones or have they been misunderstood? Look at ways of using body language, tone of voice and choice of words to enhance our messages in a positive way: for example, 'Have I understood what you said correctly?' 'Do you mean ... ?'

WORDS 2

Aim: To recognize different interpretations of words and find ways of making intended meaning clear

Age: Adults

Time: Two to two and a half hours

Equipment: Paper, pens, display board

■ Activity

1 Individuals in the group write down on a sheet of paper one word that describes how they are feeling at the present time. They fold and pass these pieces of paper at random around the circle.

2 Each paper in turn is opened and the word is read out loud, with the recipient stating what that word means to them. This is written down on a large sheet of paper by the trainer. The person who wrote the word then explains what it meant for them, which is added to the sheet.

3 The group discusses the different interpretations and explores any emotions that individuals felt had affected delivery and interpretation of the words. The trainer develops this understanding by reflecting on physical feelings and thoughts that are present before, during or after delivery of a word. Eventually a list is made of various meanings and possible feelings behind their delivery.

4 Once understanding is attained regarding emotions that can affect our use of words, the trainer can link this to the physical message of body language, by reflecting on and demonstrating how the body language can change the meaning of the word for the user and the recipient.

5 Working in pairs, participants choose one of the words and role-play (this includes body language) two possible interpretations. (They can sit or stand to do this.) They feed back and demonstrate to the group.

6 The group discusses the importance of recognizing an individual's ability to enhance comprehension by exploring the benefits of releasing tension and feeling relaxed when using words or receiving them. They look at our personal interpretations of words used by others and see whether

changing these reduces the likelihood of misinterpretation and tension.

7 Pairs experiment to see whether altering body language, tone of voice, volume, speed of delivery and thoughts of the receiver impairs or enhances the effect of the word. This is followed by feed back and demonstration to the group, and evaluation.

WORDS 3

Aim: To recognize that we can use words to enhance our beliefs in our ability to relax ourselves

Age: Teenagers/adults

Time: 90 minutes

Equipment: Large sheets of paper with sentences written on them

■ Activity

1 Reflection and discussion on previous session ('Words 2'). Exploration of what participants have learnt, how they perceived themselves and others and any subsequent positive or negative changes that have been noticed.

2 Look at the phrases people use when thinking about themselves: for example, 'I'm useless', 'I look terrible', 'I feel great today, I can achieve anything', 'I'm too old for this', 'They think I am stupid'. Make a list of sentences the group members use to praise or belittle themselves or of those others often use to them.

3 Reflect on the meanings and emotions behind these sentences and in particular specific words that enhance or diminish their self-belief. The trainer asks questions that establish the evidence behind the statements previously made (often misinterpreted). The trainer gives examples of sentences that can help an individual to cope: 'I do not have to do this, there is no gun at my head. If I do it, I am choosing to do so. Therefore I am in control'; 'They know I am capable of doing my work, even when I make a mistake'; 'I can stand making mistakes, I learn from them.'

4 In pairs, participants work together trying to change the receiver's destructive thought patterns into realistic ones. (The trainer takes on a peripatetic role here, sitting and listening — discreetly — to each couple, offering advice if necessary.)

5 Feedback from pairs is shared with the group, followed by evaluation of the session and ways to change perceptions of specific sentences using constructive thought processes and body language.

WORDS 4

Aim: To recognize the control we can have over the words we use, their delivery and reception by others
Age: Teenagers/adults
Time: 60 to 90 minutes
Equipment: Large sheets of paper, word cards, mats

■ Activity

1   The group sits in a circle, on mats. One person picks up a word card and reads it out, saying what they think it means, passing it to another person who tries to give another meaning of the word, and so on until no other meaning is found or the card has been all the way round the circle. All answers are written up on a sheet of paper. The trainer needs to use words suitable for the age group, which could have been established in an earlier session, highlighting words often used by them.

2   Discussion of the different words and their possible meanings. Do body language and tone of voice alter the meaning?

3   One person role-plays a word without saying what it is and the others try to guess it. Who was right (if anyone)? What clues were given?

4   Working in pairs, one participant acts out a word and chooses an emotion to go with it, such as anger, frustration, or sadness, and the other guesses what the word is and what emotion was linked to it.

5   Pairs demonstrate to the group, who try to guess the emotion displayed. This leads to recognition that emotion can change a word's meaning and the way it is perceived by another person.

■ Development

Look at situations in which the group recognize that the emotion may have changed the meaning of the word either for themselves or for the person receiving it. Positive ways of changing the body language and use of words in order to promote clarity, comprehension and ease for both parties. (Teenagers like this as they are able to role-play ways of dealing with difficult situations associated with puberty.)

MAIN THEME

WORDS 5

Aim: To clarify understanding of personal control that can be achieved by reflecting on body language, voice and words
Age: Teenagers/adults
Time: 60–90 minutes
Equipment: Paper, pen, board

■ Activity

1 Reflection on the previous session. A reminder of the importance of body language, delivery, pitch, tone, volume and emotion when we give or receive messages via the spoken word.

2 Group discussion of situations in which individuals feel they have been misunderstood or got their message across. A list is made by the trainer.

3 In pairs, participants choose a situation to role-play from the examples given, aiming to enact the situation in the way that was described. One person relays the message as they thought it was delivered, the other reacts to it in the way they feel they would have done.

4 Demonstration by each couple to the group is followed by general discussion, with reflections from the group about what the message was, how it was received and what, if anything, could be changed. The group divides into pairs again to try out the changes and see if any altered feelings result.

5 Feedback on any differences: the trainer highlights the way emotions can change perceptions, and indicates ways of relieving these emotions so that a person can feel more in control.

■ Development

Look at specific situations that individuals are nervous of having to deal with and seek positive ways of handling them. Situations might include: going for an interview; facing a colleague when emotions have been running high and calmly explaining how they feel; or talking to a teacher when they feel they have been criticized with or without reason.

WORDS 6

Aim: To instil recognition that individuals can control the way they speak and the words they choose to use

Age: Teenagers/adults

Time: 30–90 minutes

Equipment: Word cards

■ Activity

1   Sitting in a circle, participants take turns in picking a card, spelling and then reading out the word.

2   The group explores the meanings of the words, acting out these meanings in movement (fast, slow, hot, cold, tight, loose and so on), seeing that sometimes you can show a word's meaning without saying it.

3   The group works on recognizing that bodily movements and the way we say the words add to the meaning. For example, each person has to show the word 'dig' when angry, when happy and when sad.

4   Demonstration by half the group while the other half watch: the watchers state what emotions they feel are being shown. Then roles are reversed.

5   The group discusses the ways we give messages to people when we want to receive something or to reject someone who denies us what we want.

6   Pairs role-play in movement, drama and voice situations where one person asks for something and the other first agrees and then says 'no'. Pairs demonstrate to the group. Participants discuss how they felt, what their body and voice were like, how the words came out.

7   Looking at ways of changing the responses of both parties, the trainer demonstrates how to ask for things in a way that is not full of tension and anxiety, and how to accept the word 'no' without feeling rejected.

8   Original pairs practise these techniques and see how it feels. They then feed back to the group.

MAIN THEME

SENTENCES

Aim: To explore the use of phrases that individuals believe in as a means of encouraging deep relaxation
Age: Adults
Time: One to two hours
Equipment: Mats and pillows, paper and pens

■ Activity

1   In a circle, individuals discuss their ability to relax themselves and the theory and practice of using particular phrases to enhance a relaxed state.

2   Group discussion and compilation of phrases that are conducive to relaxation.

3   Practice of relaxation in a chair (see pages 38–9) enhanced by the use of the phrases. General discussion of how everybody felt: their likes and dislikes.

4   Practice of a short relaxation technique to be used at work or at home when feeling pressure. Individuals close their eyes and repeat calming phrases as they breathe comfortably. For example:

I feel tired and heavy	repeated twice
The heaviness is leaving me	repeated 3 times
I feel warm	repeated 4 times
I feel calmer	repeated 5 times
I can cope with this situation	repeated 6 times (can be linked with visualization of themselves coping)

5   In pairs, participants work on creating phrases that they feel enable them to enter a relaxed state.

6   Feedback: participants read out their phrases. Everyone practices these phrases closing their eyes, breathing deeply five times, allowing their bodies to go soft and then repeating the phrases as spoken by the particular pair. The group as a whole evaluates each phrase. They establish which phrases everyone likes.

7   Review of the purpose of the session.

8   Full relaxation, adding in phrases from stage 5, each one repeated three times.

9   Feedback and evaluation of the session.

BREATHING TECHNIQUES 1

Aim: To provide theoretical information and evidence of the benefits of breathing techniques to induce or enhance a relaxed state

Age: Teenagers/adults

Time: 90–120 minutes

Equipment: Large display sheets or overhead projector

■ Activity

1 With the group sitting in a circle, the trainer establishes understanding of the way we breathe, problems we may encounter and benefits derived from using the lungs properly (see pages 26–7). The trainer lists any problems identified by the group.

2 Group interaction: individuals place one hand on the upper chest and the other below the rib cage to establish which moves as they breathe; practice of diaphragmatic breathing (see pages 29–30); discussion of how participants feel and any problems, such as hyperventilation.

3 Looking at situations in which individuals have felt or feel anxious, ways of feeling calmer are expressed. Using an example given by a group member, the trainer asks the individual to close their eyes and visualize the scene, explaining how they feel as they do so; they are encouraged to take deep breaths as the situation develops and particularly before they speak. Discussion follows on any changes that occurred. *Note*: the trainer here is responsible for making the visualization relevant to the person, feeding the situation by verbalizing aspects that the individual has already told the group about. Everyone tries out this technique.

4 After feedback and evaluation of the session's activity, participants are given the home task of practising the deep breathing technique once a day, either while sitting down or just before an expected difficult situation occurs, such as a train being delayed and making them late for work, writing down after each occasion how they felt and any changes that occurred. These notes are to be brought with them to the next session.

BREATHING TECHNIQUES 2

Aim: To clarify uses and benefits of breathing techniques in everyday situations and when linked to relaxation

Age: Teenagers/adults

Time: 90–120 minutes

■ Activity

1 Breathing techniques and relaxation (sitting) are used to warm up the group (see pages 44–5). The group then shares experiences from the previous session, its practice and any outcome.

2 They continue to look at their list of specific issues that have felt difficult or are now apparent. Working in pairs, they talk through these issues, establishing how they feel now and whether they breathe more deeply. Feedback to the group follows.

3 The trainer begins to work on the link between body language and tension, which is heightened by shallow breathing. The trainer asks for examples from group members of situations in which they have felt tense and recognize the body language of another person.

4 In pairs, participants choose one of these situations and role-play it, going straight through it once and then, a second time, trying to take a deep breath before they speak or answer the other person. Feedback and demonstrations are followed by group discussion of what changes in body language were apparent when they consciously breathed: did it help?

5 The trainer gets everyone to walk around the room breathing comfortably, then deeply, stretching their arms up above their heads as they do so, then breathing normally.

6 Pairs perform the role-plays, again with the emphasis on changing body language and on comfortable breathing with occasional deep breaths. Feedback, demonstrations and discussion follow as before. Did the forced break of movement and breathing make the role-play more comfortable? How could participants use this idea in the future as a means of preparing to deal with a situation that they know may occur?

BREATHING TECHNIQUES 3

Aim: To recognize that exercise will be more enjoyable, and easier to do, when linked with appropriate breathing skills

Age: Teenagers/adults

Time: 90 minutes

Equipment: Gym or large hall, mats, benches, balls, hoops, circuit work-out sheets

■ Activity

1   Following warm-up, participants sit in a circle around a particular mat. The trainer demonstrates the correct way to complete an exercise, making clear when to breathe in and when to breathe out. Everyone tries out the right and the wrong way to breathe (see pages 29–30).

2   Discussion of the differences correct breathing generates.

3   Moving on to different pieces of apparatus, the trainer gives clear demonstrations of exercise and the natural breathing rhythm that will enhance performance. For example, as the number of step-ups increases, so more oxygen is needed and therefore deeper breaths are necessary. Everyone practises.

4   This continues around all the set tasks until all the activities have been demonstrated by the trainer and practised by group members and the most efficient breathing pattern has been established.

5   A timed or numbered circuit of exercises for the whole group. *Note*: always start with low numbers, before moving on to higher ones. Use the numbered approach before the timed circuit as individuals will often forget the breathing patterns needed in order to finish within the set time.

6   Participants cool down by walking around the room, slowly, increasing depth of breath until the heart rate slows down and they feel calm. Finish with relaxation (see 'Relax Down 12').

BREATHING TECHNIQUES 4

Aim: To understand and use breathing techniques to enhance a relaxed state

Age: Teenagers/adults

Time: 45 minutes

■ Activity

1 The trainer reiterates the importance of relaxation and the understanding of tension and release.

2 The seated relaxation technique (see pages 38–9) is practised, first without and then with conscious breathing. Discussion of the differences experienced follows.

3 The trainer emphasizes that it is not necessary to tense in order to release and then the group practise relaxation using breathing and thought process.

4 Discussion of situations when people are sitting, in which they could use the above technique and then enhance this practice with positive statements (see page 31).

5 Feedback, discussion and evaluation of breathing techniques to create control and calmness.

6 Full relaxation as for 'Relax Down 2'. (See also pages 38–9)

STRESS MANAGEMENT 1

Aim: To recognize, understand and seek ways of coping with areas of stress

Age: Teenagers/adults

Time: Two to two and a half hours

Equipment: Large (A3) sheets of paper with information on the workshop, or an overhead projector

■ Activity

1 With the group in a circle, sitting on chairs, the trainer establishes with questions and answers what stress is, what stress management is and what stress means to individuals.

2 The trainer provides a worksheet or overhead projection that highlights possible physical, emotional, behavioural and mental signs that indicate stress in individuals. The group use this to establish how stress shows itself in their lives, highlighting the major examples. They discuss and share these stresses, acknowledging similarities and differences.

3 The trainer now aims to show the group ways of understanding when their level of stress is manageable and when unmanageable (see pages 55–6). Clarification is achieved by getting group members to describe situations where they feel they were and were not in control.

4 Discussion follows of ways of dealing with hitherto unmanageable stress, such as use of stability zones and rituals and places that we all use in order to cope, such as taking a bath, reading, walking on a beach or having a cup of tea while reading the paper.

5 Once such techniques have been recognized, individuals consider whether any of these stability zones and rituals could be used to lessen the impact of the identified areas of physical, emotional, behavioural and mental stress. A new list is made of the ones that need other skills.

6 Sometimes, depending on the needs of the group and the level of stress, it is expedient to teach a specific coping mechanism to the whole group. For example, if there are several people who have sleeping difficulties you could teach everyone distraction and calming techniques to use to go to sleep.

113

7 Evaluation of the session: clarifying aspects that can be dealt with and areas that at the present time cannot.

8 'Relax Down 15'.

STRESS MANAGEMENT 2

Aim: To continue to develop understanding by participants of their own ability to deal with areas of stress that feel unmanageable

Age: Teenagers/adults

Time: Two to two and a half hours

Equipment: Large (A3) sheets of paper with information on the workshop, or an overhead projector

■ Activity

1   After a relaxation warm-up focusing on creating comfort and empathy, the group reflect on the previous session, in particular any areas where stress has been reduced or is still prevalent.

2   A list of all the major stresses, as identified at the previous session, is displayed, plus any additions that have come to light over the past week.

3   The trainer uses a worksheet or overhead projection to help individuals to recognize their own abilities that they use subconsciously or consciously to get them through difficult situations. For example, they may talk to someone, accept their own limitations, listen or delegate.

4   The group look at ways of using these abilities to reduce their identified stresses.

5   The group prioritize their major stresses into a list to be worked through over the next few sessions to find coping skills, starting with tension and the benefits of the use of relaxation as a means of reducing its impact.

6   'Relax Down 1' and 'Relax Down 2'.

7   Feedback and evaluation.

STRESS MANAGEMENT 3

Aim: To continue the process of establishing coping mechanisms that individuals can choose to use to relieve what has been unmanageable stress

Age: Teenagers/adults

Time: Two to two and a half hours

■ Activity

1 Review of the previous session. The content of this workshop is dependent on the needs highlighted by the group in the previous two sessions. Some guidelines to help you with certain issues will be found on pages 53–6.

2 The group looks at the benefits of breathing techniques to reduce stress (as for 'Breathing techniques 1', but in a simplified form).

3 Participants highlight identified tension created by pressure and examples from their list of physical, emotional, behavioural and mental symptoms which would benefit from a breathing technique. They practise this technique while sitting.

4 After relaxation while sitting, participants are encouraged to visualize situations that have caused them stress and, using the breathing technique, to seek to alter the physical and emotional symptoms that are experienced.

5 Feedback and discussion of situations in which individuals feel they could use this breathing technique to reduce their stress.

STRESS MANAGEMENT 4

Aim: To enable individuals to focus on the importance of dealing with, rather than avoiding, situations in order to reduce their level of stress and to help them feel in control

Age: Teenagers/adults

Time: Two to two and a half hours

■ Activity

1 Review of the previous session, any changes that have occurred, and any problems, highlighting the area of identified stress to be dealt with in the present session.

2 Discussion of avoidance: what it does, how it affects the body, mind and behaviour; the benefits of challenging avoidance.

3 Ways of dealing with avoidance. The trainer encourages participants to share experiences where they recognize they have avoided rather than dealt with a problem. The trainer offers guidance on ways to deal with a situation that has been highlighted by a group member and in which they avoided rather than dealt with a situation. Working in pairs, participants role-play this situation.

4 Each pair demonstrates how they would seek to deal with the problem. The group discusses these demonstrations and decides on a technique that will be helpful to everyone. They then practise this in pairs and feed back to the group how it felt. Participants say whether they personally would use this technique.

5 Participants' homework is to seek to deal with, rather than avoid, situations. A notebook is to be kept in which they write down instances of dealing with or avoiding a situation, feelings at the time and afterwards, to be brought to the next session.

6 'Relax Down 16'; with participants seeing themselves in a situation where they face the problem and deal with it: calmly, feeling good, in control.

STRESS MANAGEMENT 5

Aim: To establish that an individual can never be a complete failure, that failure is a way of learning that is a natural part of our lives

Age: Teenagers/adults

Time: Two to two and a half hours

Equipment: Paper, pens, pencils

■ Activity

1   Warm up using a relaxation technique that encourages empathy and willingness to be open. Review the previous session and, where necessary, reiterate or clarify the skill that had been learnt. Highlight the area of stress to be dealt with in that present session.

2   Explore the word failure, its realistic and emotional meanings.

3   Make a list of times when individuals feel they have failed. Using an example given by the group, the trainer asks questions to establish evidence of failure that inevitably shows that the failure was not total.

4   Taking the initial of their first name and drawing it on a piece of paper, participants write inside it everything about themselves. They share this information with the group, highlighting any area where they feel a failure.

5   The trainer disputes this failure by reminding them that, as failure is total, absolute and they have only highlighted some aspects of themselves, they cannot be a total failure. They may have failed in one aspect, but only one, and, if they have learnt from it, then even it has become a partial success.

■ Development

1   Highlight the area in which each person considers themselves a failure, using a technique that lists good and bad aspects about this failure. Challenge the bad aspects by highlighting grey areas, establish the good aspects as positive qualities, then deal with the aspects that need change (usually to do with self-worth). Encourage group participation in finding ways of dealing with the remaining issue or issues.

2 'Relax Down 17': use the sentences provided or make up others with the group.

3 Feedback and evaluation.

■ Note

In order for trainers to work effectively with this theme they need to have some understanding, belief and training in Cognitive Behavioural Therapy, a concept often explored in stress management courses.

STRESS MANAGEMENT 6

Aim: To help individuals to recognize the power of their own minds to alter their physical state
Age: Teenagers/adults
Time: Two to two and a half hours

■ Activity

1 Review the previous session, good and bad practice by individuals and any aspect that needs clarification.
2 Explore the issues of hypnosis and self-hypnosis, clarifying the differences between stage and professional therapy and statements of self-belief.
3 Look at the power of the mind and its ability to alter our physical state. For example, thinking "I can't stand it", which can lead to apathy, tension and panic, may be changed to "I don't have to do this, I am choosing to, therefore I can stand it", which releases tension, calms the person and enhances feelings of being in control.
4 Discuss situations where negative thoughts have resulted in negative emotions. Encourage each person to give an example. Use these examples to demonstrate that, by using realistic positive statements (as detailed above) participants can alter the physical and emotional effects of negative beliefs.
5 Individuals practice relaxation in chairs, then focus on the situation described by them, first repeating in their minds their previous negative thoughts, recognizing the tension aroused, then using the constructive, realistic phrases they have learnt, seeing whether they release this tension. Feedback and group discussion on the outcomes follow.
6 'Relax Down 14'.

■ Note

In order for trainers to work effectively with this theme they need to have some understanding, belief and training in Rational Emotive Therapy, a concept often explored in stress management courses.

STRESS MANAGEMENT 7

Aim: To look at individuals' physical symptoms of stress that can be alleviated by the use of stress management techniques
Age: Teenagers/adults
Time: Two to two and a half hours

■ Activity

1 A review of the previous session, with an update on personal coping skills and practice, and evaluation of changes made. The area of physical stresses to be dealt with in the present session is highlighted.

2 Discussion of the physical symptoms of stress felt by individuals in the group, such as tension, headaches, nausea, diarrhoea, constipation, panic attacks, palpitations, sleeplessness, backache or cramps.

3 Exploring when the symptoms occur: before, during or after a stressful situation or at a time that has no relevance to the symptom.

4 The trainer establishes through discussion that the symptoms detailed by individuals are a physical reaction to an emotion, also known as a 'core belief'. The trainer explains that, as this core belief can trigger a physical symptom, challenging and changing this core belief can also reduce or eradicate it.

5 Look at ways in which individuals can deal with the symptoms: for example, breathing techniques, exercise, relaxation, challenging thoughts, distraction techniques, massage, change of diet or eating habits, taking time for themselves.

6 Full relaxation with breathing to reduce tension, together with the use of phrases such as "Now I am relaxed, I feel more able to deal with the issue that is causing my symptom" (individuals state what the issue is and the physical symptom it encourages) or of music to enhance the relaxed state.

STRESS MANAGEMENT 8

Aim: To enable individuals to reflect on the importance of self-worth, to acknowledge and build upon their qualities, rather than dwell on their believed inadequacies

Age: Teenagers/adults

Time: Two to two and a half hours

Equipment: Pens and paper

■ Activity

1 A review of the previous session, with clarification of the issues that were dealt with, and examples of practice and changes that have occurred.

2 Highlighting the importance of how participants feel about themselves, the trainer establishes that, when we like ourselves, we work better, our relationships are better, we feel good. When we feel bad we see faults in everything we or others do; we can be subject to feelings of rejection, persecution and inadequacy.

3 Participants write a list of the positive and negative aspects of themselves and then explain these views to their partners.

4 Feedback to the group is followed by discussion of these views: is there evidence to support them? Using a volunteer, the trainer establishes a pattern of destructive thoughts that are not based on logic but on emotions; enables the person concerned to work through a process of self-acknowledgement, highlighting qualities, focusing on the core element, such as fear of failure; and helping the individual to recognize ways of coping with and altering the effects of their destructive beliefs through practical as well as thought-challenging processes.

5 In pairs, participants review their lists and see if they can challenge their own beliefs and alter any of the negatives. They then come back to the group with any aspects that they still identify as negative.

6 The trainer reviews each person's 'negative' aspect and offers ways of changing this to an aspect that is more acceptable to the individual.

■ Development

1   If there are couples present, you could work on relationship issues by encouraging them to write a positive and negative list not only about themselves, but also about each other. (This is often much more positive than it may at first seem likely to be.)

2   Relaxation with breathing techniques and thoughts of self-worth to encourage individuals to like and accept themselves.

STRESS MANAGEMENT 9

Aim: To reflect on the negative aspects of having unrealistic
goals that are causing unnecessary stress and to clarify ways
of changing this stress by using achievable short-term goals

Age: Teenagers/adults

Time: Two to two and a half hours

Equipment: Pens and paper

■ Activity

1   A review of the previous session, coping mechanisms found
and, if they were used, the results — both good and bad.

2   The trainer asks the group to reflect on goals they have for the
next year, five years, 10 years. A list is made.

3   Each person chooses just one goal they would like to attain and
writes down what this entails. They share this with other group
members.

4   Once clarity about personal goals is achieved, individuals can
be relaxed (while sitting) and asked to picture themselves
achieving their desired goal: how do they feel? Is it what they
wanted?

5   The trainer establishes the importance of goals that are
achievable, an effective stress management tool of seeing goals
in stages, using checklists that provide evidence of success
while highlighting areas of failure that can be reviewed and
used as a stepping-stone to achievement of the goal.

6   Relaxation with imagery, as before, but this time seeing
themselves achieving a stage of the goal, clarifying how they
feel and any problems they have thought of or experienced.
Feedback and general discussion follows.

7   Review of the session. For homework, individuals go away and
think about what is their real goal, how it can be achieved and
in what stages. They are to list all these, practising the
relaxation with imagery and bring the results to the next session
to share with the group.

STRESS MANAGEMENT 10

Aim: To seek to understand the destructive ways we use words
that create tension and lack of self-worth
Age: Teenagers/adults
Time: Two to two and a half hours

■ Activity

1 Review of the previous session and overview of coping
   mechanisms that have been learnt throughout the course.
2 Discussion of our use of words, in particular words such as
   'have to', 'should' and 'must', reflecting on the emotions these
   words evoke in us. The trainer asks for examples from group
   members of the way they use these words and in what contexts,
   exploring the emotions and physical feelings that are present.
3 The trainer suggests phrases that change or challenge the use
   of such words in situations that are causing anxiety: for
   example, 'I do not have to, I am choosing to'; 'Life is not fair,
   therefore all the "shoulds" in this life are "I would prefer it to
   be"'; 'People control their own behaviour and therefore when
   you are about to say to yourself "I must" say "I choose to"
   instead'; 'Often the words "I cannot cope" can be changed to "I
   can cope, I am coping all the time, I will find a way"'.
4 Feed back reactions from the group, ideas for changing or
   challenging words. The aim is to practise whenever there is
   negative use of these words.

STRESS MANAGEMENT 11

Aim: To develop self-confidence and belief in participants' abilities to present themselves well at an interview
Age: Teenagers/adults
Time: Two to two and a half hours
Equipment: Large sheet of paper, pen

■ Activity

1 Review of previous session: any thoughts, feelings or outcomes.
2 The trainer looks at specific situations in order to provide participants with coping skills, specifically those needed in an interview.
3 Discussion of the issues related to an interview, such as body language, dress, anxiety and nervousness about saying the wrong thing or the questions that will be asked. A list is made for all to see.
4 The group works through the issues and finds coping mechanisms to deal with them: breathing techniques to use before entering the room, before answering and during the answering of each question; body language — how to walk, how to sit, how to focus on one person who has asked a question and how to gain the attention of several interview panel members by moving eye contact from one to another as they answer.
5 Participants work in pairs — one as the interviewer, the other as the interviewee. They practise positive self-control techniques. The trainer can either set questions or encourage participants to make up their own. Once the role-play is over, participants swap roles.
6 Group feedback, demonstrations and discussion of good and bad practice.
7 Relaxation, sitting, as on pages 38–9, together with participants' visualization of themselves in an interview: 'Focus on the room; watch yourself enter, calmly, body erect, shoulders back, breathing comfortably. Look at the interview chair as you enter: does it need to be moved; is it too close or too far away from the interviewers? As you reach the chair, move it slightly so that you feel in control. Sit down comfortably, place your hands in a

comfortable position, smile as you are spoken to. Maintain eye contact with the person asking the question; initially reply to that person then move your eyes to respond to everyone else. Take a deep breath between replies. You are looking good, feeling good, you can answer a question without falling to pieces.'

8 Feedback from everyone. Homework is to practise in front of a mirror.

STRESS MANAGEMENT 12

Aim: To establish personal understanding of the part thoughts play in creating emotions and seeing these early warning signals by using a biofeedback machine (training is necessary before you attempt this: see Appendix)
Age: Teenagers/adults
Time: 90–120 minutes
Equipment: Biofeedback machines, pens and paper

■ Activity

1 In a circle, participants discuss fears people have of different things: dentists, doctors, lifts, trains, spiders, and so on.
2 The trainer gives a reminder of the use of breathing techniques to calm us. The group practises these.
3 Discussion of the use of biofeedback machines and their purpose. The trainer asks a volunteer to close their eyes and focus on a situation or event they dislike (not too frightening), listening to see if the sound rises. When it does, the trainer encourages them to breathe deeply but comfortably and see the fear diminish.
4 In the subsequent discussion, the trainer shows that thoughts create emotions. There follows a review of phrases that individuals in the group tend to use about their fear, looking at the truth or otherwise of these and seeking new phrases that are constructive, realistic challenges to the old and that reduce tension.
5 Working in pairs (several machines are needed for this) participants establish what their fear is, writing it down, discussing phrases that can challenge the fear and that are believed by the individual. One person then closes their eyes and visualizes their fear while attached to the machine. When the sound rises their partner reads out the phrases, which are repeated mentally by the visualizer, who also breathes deeply. When the sound falls they open their eyes. *The trainer needs to be observant here*: if a sound is not diminishing, they need to take over and provide the thought challenges to reduce the individual's anxiety.
6 Feedback, exploration of the session, clarification of its purpose and outcome.

STRESS MANAGEMENT 13

Aim: To encourage personal understanding by the use of biodots, of the way body temperatures rise when we feel stressed

Age: Teenagers/adults

Time: 20 minutes

Equipment: Biodots, pens, paper

■ Activity

1   The group discuss previous use of biofeedback or bodily messages that provide signals or signs of tension and stress.

2   Explain the use of biodots: there are two types, low and high temperature. Give both types to each individual. They are to press the dot, holding it for 10 seconds, then releasing it and seeing what colour is shown. They then read the chart and see what it says. Discussion follows: has the result surprised them, or were they already aware of their feelings?

3   Explore their understanding and any signals they recognize in their bodies.

4   Use a relaxation technique (sitting), with participants pressing their dots before they begin and writing down the results. On completing the relaxation, they press their dots again and write down the findings. Feedback and clarification of any changes follow.

5   Use a relaxation technique (lying), with participants pressing their dots before and after the relaxation, noting any changes. Feedback: how clearly do participants understand their own ability to alter the way they feel by using relaxation techniques?

■ Development

This is a good way of introducing a theme on relaxation or of demonstrating control of stress during another session.

MAIN THEME

SELF-WORTH

Aim: To help individuals to come to terms with loss and recognition of loss as a natural process as well as their own ability to lessen its impact

Age: Teenagers/adults

Time: Two to three hours

Equipment: Large sheet of paper, pen

■ Activity

1 Discussion of the issues and levels of loss that there are: for example, loss of friend, job, family, partner (through death, rejection or their moving away), as well as loss of opportunity (as with couples wanting a child).

2 The trainer compiles a list of all the 'losses' identified by the group and establishes that loss can be momentary or sustained.

3 The group looks at ways of helping themselves to grieve and release emotions and the difficulties created by withholding them. Ways of helping include recognizing that they have a right to grieve; letting others know what they are grieving for and telling them they do not need to do anything; allowing themselves to cry if they want to, telling others to let them do so, and not to try to 'bring them out of it'; talking through feelings with others who have experienced the same loss or with a trained counsellor who can enable a person to clarify, understand and deal with their emotions; changing thoughts about themselves that are negative and destructive into ones that are realistic, accepting themselves warts and all, and which offer comfort and hope.

4 The group discusses the use of relaxation and breathing techniques (practising them) particularly once emotion has been released.

5 Practice of relaxation and breathing techniques linked to full relaxation. Feedback and evaluation.

130

ALTERNATIVE THERAPIES

Aim: To introduce participants to other avenues of relaxation using alternative therapies (see Appendix for details of other therapies)

Age: Adult

Time: Two hours

Equipment: Pencils

■ Activity

1   Discussion on the use of an alternative therapy, such as acupuncture, its aims and objectives. Has anyone tried it? Does anyone wish to do so?

2   The group discusses the fear of needles, highlighting ways individual participants cope with it. The discussion is then broadened to encompass all coping techniques.

3   Working in pairs, participants take it in turns to close their eyes, visualize a needle and say how they feel and where tension is felt. They take several deep breaths and see if this reduces the tension. They visualize the needle leaving the body.

4   Group discussion: how did participants feel?

5   The trainer offers ideas for coping with needles, such as taking several deep breaths, wiggling their toes, closing their eyes or focusing on something pleasant.

6   Working in pairs, one person sits ready to receive a 'pretend' needle (a pencil — not the sharp end). They practise wiggling their toes, breathing deeply, saying when they are ready. Partners then change over and repeat. Partners discuss how it felt. Changing over again, this time they use the sharp end of the 'needle' to touch the skin. Then they change over for the last time.

7   Feedback and discussion with the group: any changes, any problems still present?

8   Relaxation with imagery (see pages 40–1): 'Focusing on a needle; seeing yourself coping comfortably, saying when you are ready; looking at the needle and seeing how small it is; looking away or focusing on it as it nears the body; wiggling the toes and fingers, breathing deeply, counting to 10 slowly. It is all over. You feel good: you were in control. You can stand it.'

ART

Aim: To show individuals that art can be a way of releasing pent-up emotions, enabling control to take place
Age: Teenagers/adults
Time: Two hours
Equipment: Paper, pens, crayons, paints

■ Activity

1 Participants are relaxed by the trainer on entering to encourage receptiveness to working in the workshop format.
2 Discussion of areas of tension that are now being felt: where they are in the body, how participants feel and how they felt when they entered.
3 Exploration of the use of art to explore this tension. Encourage individuals to take a sheet of paper and any medium they like to a space on the floor. They draw a picture of what the tension looks like in their bodies. (You could get them to visualize it first.)
4 In pairs, they explain to partners what the picture is saying.
5 They feed back to the whole group, sharing the picture, exploring, saying whether the tension still feels the same. Recognition of the importance of releasing feelings.
6 Discussion of this remaining tension: what is its cause — the trainer uses constructive thoughts to challenge individuals' beliefs. Each person closes their eyes, focusing on the tension, and uses the suggested thoughts to help them picture the tension changing its shape and colour, and then to redraw the picture as they now see it.
7 Individuals feed back to the whole group. Evaluation of the use of art as a means of expression.
8 'Relax Down 7'.

BODY ALIGNMENT 1

Aim: To establish awareness of good and bad posture
Age: Teenagers/adults
Time: Two hours
Equipment: A full-length mirror, paper, pencils

■ Activity

1   Walking around the room, each time participants pass the mirror they look at themselves.

2   Working in pairs, one sits or stands in their normal way, while the other draws an outline of their body shape. They change over and repeat. Pairs discuss what they saw, how they can change to a position that has better alignment and is still comfortable.

3   Each pair demonstrates their first and changed postures. After a general group discussion of the changes, the trainer elicits examples of uncomfortable postures and then demonstrates effective ways of changing them to good postures.

4   The group explores body positions that are linked to our emotions (see pages 13–14). Individuals who recognize some of these traits in themselves explore ways of changing, using breathing techniques to release tension, together with realistic challenges to damning thoughts.

5   Relaxation, emphasizing the importance of body alignment, releasing and stretching out the limbs (see pages 38–9).

6   Feedback and evaluation of the session. For homework, participants are to watch how others move, practising good alignment (see pages 17–19).

BODY ALIGNMENT 2

Aim: To recognize that we can alter our posture through
     stretching and relaxing exercises
Age: Teenagers/adults
Time: Two to two and a half hours
Equipment: Mats, bean-bags

■ **Activity**
1   Reflection on how participants feel, what they have noticed
    others do and ways they have actually tried to alter an
    emotional state by changing their body position.
2   The group is split into two. Group B watch as group A walk
    across the room together. They then walk back again, focusing
    their eyes on a particular spot. The groups swop over and
    repeat. Discussion follows on the differences noticed in body
    alignment when a focal point is used.
       Group B watch as group A (well spaced out) put on
    blindfolds and walk eight steps, remove the blindfolds and see
    where they are. The groups change over and repeat. The
    whole group then discusses the need to listen to the body.
    A bean-bag placed on the head could also be used to
    encourage an upright stance while walking.
3   The trainer lists the benefits of exercise (see pages 49–50),
    exploring ways in which exercise can enhance good posture,
    and emphasizes the need to loosen up the body with a simple
    warm-up before stretching.

134

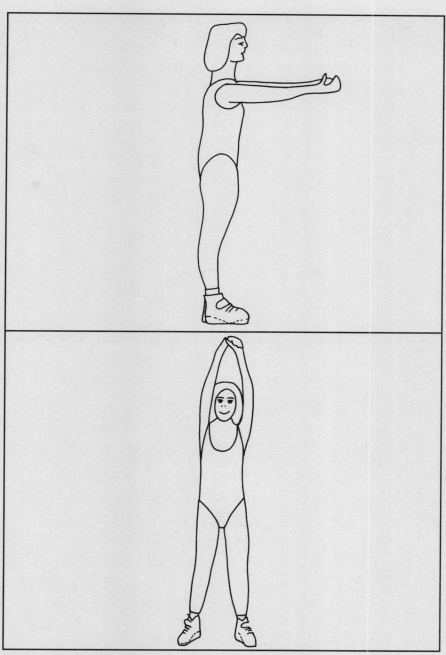

Shoulder stretches

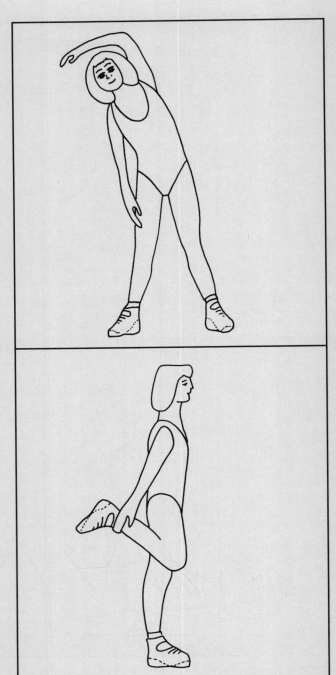

Sideways stretch

Thigh stretch

136

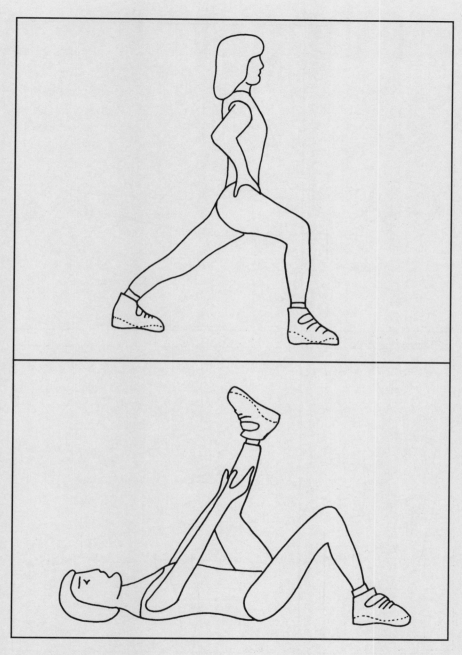

Calf stretches

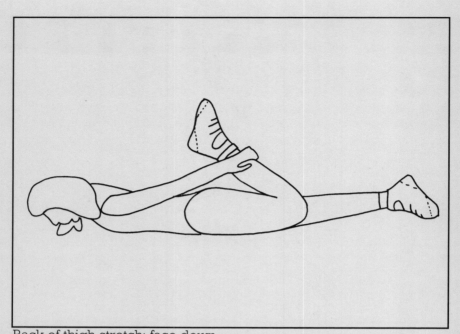

Back of thigh stretch: face down

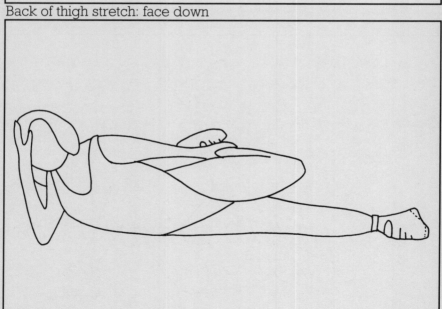

Back of thigh stretch: on side

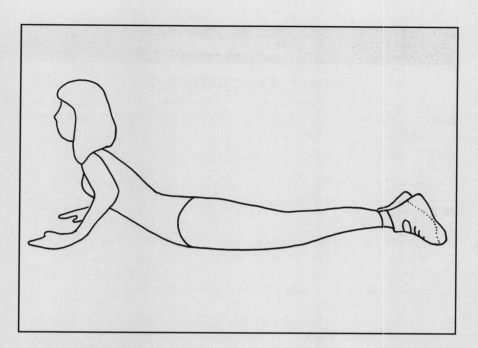

Stomach stretch

4 The trainer asks how the participants felt.
5 Relaxation (see pages 38–9) followed by phrases about stretching to enhance the relaxed state: for example, 'Feel the body stretching out as you breathe out and relax.'
6 As homework, participants are to practise every day, ensuring they warm up first (holding stretches for eight seconds only).

BODY ALIGNMENT 3

Aim: To develop the individual's ability to alter their posture and change the way they feel

Age: Teenagers/adults

Time: Two hours

Equipment: Paper, pen

■ Activity

1 Discussion of previous session 'Body alignment 2'. Review of individuals' practice: any problems, any differences felt.

2 The group looks at emotions, such as sadness, anger or fear. The trainer demonstrates and asks others to demonstrate the body position that they tend to assume when subject to particular emotions.

3 The trainer establishes what participants' thoughts are likely to be and makes a list of them. The point is made that the negative thoughts are heightening the individual's feelings and bad posture. The trainer emphasizes that it is thoughts that are creating the emotions, not the situation.

4 Individually or in pairs, participants practise challenging negative thoughts with positive realistic ones, at the same time using breathing techniques and changing the body position into a comfortable one.

5 Relaxation: 'Relax Down 13'.

BODY ALIGNMENT 4

Aim: To encourage teenagers to feel good about their bodies
and to recognize ways of enhancing this feeling by the way
they hold themselves

Age: Teenagers

Time: 30–60 minutes

Equipment: Pictures

■ Activity

1   Sitting in a circle, participants look at pictures of people in
different positions: squatting, sitting, standing, walking and so
on. They comment on some that are very straight and others
that look bent.

2   Participants walk around the room, tall, then bent, then twisted.
They walk as if they are soldiers, then lions.

3   They discuss how they felt, what was comfortable and what was
not. They look at the way animals are made and why they move
differently from us. It is concluded that our upright position
gives us control and feels the most comfortable.

4   Sitting on the floor, behind a desk and standing as if waiting for
a bus, participants explore the differences, changing body
positions to feel comfortable and able to listen. Individuals
demonstrate to the rest of the group. What looks good and in
control? What does not?

5   Everyone takes a deep breath, lifting their heads, smiling and
feeling good. Walking around the room, each time they meet
someone they stand still and smile, with a slight nod of the
head.

BODY ALIGNMENT 5

Aim: To continue the process of understanding our bodies and the way emotions play a part in our posture

Age: Teenagers/adults

Time: 30–90 minutes

■ Activity

1   Participants walk around the room, feeling tall, happy, smiling whenever they meet someone.

2   Discussion of the way we hold ourselves when we are sad, angry, upset, laughing, feeling unwanted or turning away from someone else. The trainer demonstrates and then asks others to try it.

3   Everyone tries to depict (in any order) each of the emotions, using the body shape that they feel would go with it. Then half the group demonstrates, while the other half watches, trying to determine which emotion is being shown. Then they change over.

4   The group talks about these emotions and whether changing their body shape, when they are sad, for example, will alter the feeling inside them. The trainer demonstrates and then everyone tries this. Feedback and discussion follow.

5   Looking at times when they feel they have been unwanted by others, how do participants react, and what does this show? The group discusses the way in which changing the body shape can alter the interpretation of others and help them to feel less distressed. (This is a useful tool where teenagers are afraid of others.)

AROMAS 1

Aim: To promote awareness of aromas that can be used to enhance relaxation
Age: Adults
Time: One hour
Equipment: A variety of aromas, paper and pen

■ Activity

This workshop is shown in two parts, but the trainer could make it one two-hour workshop by ensuring that, at the end of a previous session, the group members were told to bring along a smell they like and dislike.

Part one

1 Discussion of the uses of aromatherapy, encouraging group participation. The trainer gives information on where to find out more about it.
2 The trainer brings in some smells that they like and dislike, such as perfume, polish, spices, flowers or bread, and explains what they are and what they contain (in case of allergies). They are passed round, and the feelings of others are discussed.
3 Discussion of smells the group like. A list is made of all of them. Common and uncommon substances are commented upon.
4 Relaxation (five minutes) using an aromatic candle to see if it induces relaxation or hinders it for particular individuals. Discussion.
5 The homework task for participants is to bring in one smell that they like and one that they dislike. (*no dangerous substances* such as bleach).
6 Full relaxation, using the candle (if the whole group liked it) or 'Relax Down 8'.

■ Development

Part two

1 This session explores the smells that each person has brought in and their uses. Participants try them out as individuals and as a group.
2 The group looks at situations at work and at home where an aromatic smell would help to reduce tension and emotional feelings, such as in the bath or while working.

AROMAS 2

Aim: To stimulate memories for elderly confused people
Age: Elderly
Time: 30 minutes
Equipment: Items that were in use during the earlier lifetime of individuals, particularly when they were children

■ Activity

1 Having previously established the backgrounds of individuals by talking to a family member or the individual themselves, the trainer brings in items that could stimulate individuals' memories, such as tins containing tobacco, perfumes, soaps and flowers. (Age Concern will be helpful here.)

2 Each individual is invited to feel and smell the object, exploring the memory it jogs, and sharing that memory with the rest of the group. If members are unable to tell a story related to the feel or smell, the trainer needs to have in reserve several stories that can be shared.

3 The trainer invites individuals to choose an aromatic smell they like, letting them smell it, encouraging them to close their eyes as they do so, then to put down the smell and see if they can still remember it.

4 Using a relaxation technique (sitting), the trainer encourages them to remember the smell to enhance their feelings of calmness and happiness. (The trainer may need to pass the smell around in order to prompt the memory.)

IMAGERY 1

Aim: To enable individuals who are being treated for a severe
   illness to see ways of helping themselves to feel better and
   able to cope with their condition
Age: Teenagers/adults
Time: 1 hour
Equipment: Mats, pillows, comfortable chairs, paper, crayons or
   pencils

■ Activity

1   Discussion of the illnesses: where they are located, what they
   entail, treatment that is being used, and fears or anxieties.
2   Using paper and pencil (or crayons) participants draw what
   they think the ill part of their body looks like. Feedback:
   participants have time to share and reflect. What is each
   individual saying in their picture?
3   Discussion of the treatment: whether it is perceived as a
   'saviour'; the evidence that treatment would not be offered
   unless it had the possibility of alleviating the symptoms for a
   short or a long period of time; the importance of any time
   gained as 'Quality time'. Discussion of ways of achieving this
   quality, such as relaxation and breathing techniques, linked with
   imagery, changes to daily routines that prioritize the
   individual's wishes, closer or more frequent contact with loved
   ones or friends, more social time, more enjoyment time, simple
   pleasures.
4   The group looks in depth at the benefits of relaxation and, in
   particular, imagery. Discussion: is there a 'saviour' available?
   (This could be the treatment or their own belief system.) What
   does it look like? They will now draw this saviour, using colours
   if they wish to.
5   Feedback: does this drawing resemble the other one? What is
   different? How could the second conquer the first (recognizing
   that this victory may not be forever, but may give a respite from
   pain and distress)?
6   Practice of a relaxation technique (sitting or lying) focusing on
   the part that is ill, seeing the 'saviour' as they have drawn it,
   attacking or engulfing the bad and diminishing it.

7 Feedback from the group: how did the relaxation change their feelings? Did it help to make the illness more bearable? Are there problems?

8 Away from the workshop, individuals are to practise relaxation connected to breathing when in pain, using the imagery every day: before, during or after any treatment, or just when they feel like it. It is a good idea in these circumstances for the trainer to prepare a tape for each individual, detailing their thoughts about their 'saviour', using their own words, so as to reinforce their capacity to deal with their discomfort.

IMAGERY 2

Aim: To enable individuals to come to terms with the loss of a loved one

Age: Teenagers/adults

Time: 30 minutes to two hours, depending on age

■ Activity

1 Allow time for each member of the group (aim to keep it small — no more than 10) to tell the others about their loved one and what the loss means to them.

2 Reflection on emotions that are felt, such as anger, guilt, fear, rejection, depression, being unable to cope.

3 Recognition of the normality of these emotions and of the negative aspects of repressing or dwelling on them.

4 Relaxation technique (sitting) in order to calm down feelings at this time; seeing relaxation as a way of recharging batteries in order to be able to cope.

5 The trainer makes it possible for participants to talk about the nice and the not so nice aspects of the loved one, moving away from the 'saintly' or 'evil' concept that individuals can create of lost ones, and close to reality.

6 Discussion of imagery as a means of focusing on a happy memory of the person who has died, to produce comfort, warmth and even a smile. Exploration of other ways of dealing with loss, such as allowing oneself to cry, writing a letter to the person, looking at photographs and sitting back and remembering.

7 Feedback and evaluation. Exploration of participants' feelings that have become clearer and more acceptable since the beginning of the session.

IMAGERY 3

Aim: To provide evidence of positive ways for an individual to alter the way they feel about themselves

Age: Teenagers/adults

Time: 30 minutes to two hours, depending on age

■ Activity

1 Sitting in a circle, the group discusses ways people behave that they dislike.

2 Closing their eyes, they visualize someone behaving badly. What does it feel like inside? Partners role-play this behaviour, discussing what happened and what the messages were.

3 Partners feed back to the group their thoughts about the role-play, highlighting the messages they thought were being relayed and any possible misinterpretation.

4 Discussion of the ways individuals behave in a difficult situation: body language, words, tone, emotions. Discussion of ways of changing behaviour that can create calmness, a feeling of being in control, the reduction of fear, and the giving of clear messages. Partners work on changing the way the message was delivered in the first role-play. In feedback to the group, pairs say what changes, if any, occurred.

5 Relaxation and then imagery of themselves in the situation that they have already practised or one they feel they may need to deal with shortly. (This will have been established first, before the relaxation.) They see themselves delivering their message, changing any body language that might be negative and not conducive to communication.

6 Feedback and evaluation of the session; seeing positive ways of practising communication and feeling in control without aggression.

7 'Relax Down 11'.

IMAGERY 4

Aim: To see realistic goals as a useful aid to relaxation
Age: Teenagers/adults
Time: 30–60 minutes

■ Activity
1 Discussion of realistic and unrealistic goals and in particular the tensions that are caused by the latter. Seeing success as being more manageable and sustainable if envisaged in stages.
2 Each person states a goal they have and how far ahead they see it being achieved. They see an image of themselves achieving this goal: is it what they wanted?
3 Group feedback on ways of achieving these goals: making a list of all the steps; each day visualizing themselves achieving this step, until it is actually achieved, then moving on to the next one. If the step is not achieved, it is important to recognize that striving to achieve it embodies elements of success that make it possible to change the goal for one that can be achieved.
4 Homework is to try this process out, linking it with a relaxation technique that has already been learnt (see 'Relax Down 1' and 'Relax Down 2'.

■ Development
In the next session, participants reflect on their practice, feelings about their goal, any changes and any problems. Then they focus on thoughts to enhance their belief system, used with relaxation and imagery.

DANCE 1

Aim: To recognize ways of moving and changing feelings
Age: Teenagers/adults
Time: 30–60 minutes
Equipment: Taped music or musical instruments

■ Activity

1   Sitting in a circle, the group discusses how we move, going through the body parts: for example, single or double arm actions, one or both feet, one leg and the other leg, whole body movement.

2   The group practises movements of individual parts and then the whole body: waving, lifting, climbing a ladder, running, shaking, jumping, turning and twirling (spinning on the floor), and so on.

3   These same movements are practised, in slow motion and then at speed.

4   Participants discuss how each movement felt, highlighting any movements that felt uncomfortable, and establishing where tension or release of tension was needed to alter the pace of the action.

5   Participants move and react to the trainer as they read out a story that involves creeping, crawling, running, jumping, turning slowly and quickly, ending with stretching up tall and curling down small into a lying position, the reading and movements becoming slower and slower until the words almost drift away and the body is at rest.

■ Development

1   To quicken or slow the pace, use instruments such as tambourines or drums, or music with raised and lowered pitch or with diminuendos and crescendos.

2   Encourage participants to breathe slowly as they perform the slow movements, particularly the resting one at the end.

3   Use words to emphasize the relaxed state at the end, such as 'lighter and lighter', 'calmer and calmer', 'softer and softer', 'peaceful', 'comfortable', 'happy', 'relaxed'.

DANCE 2

Aim: To recognize the expressive use of dance to explore and release emotions, leading to a more relaxed state
Age: Teenagers/adults
Time: 45–90 minutes
Equipment: Music

■ Activity

1 Practice of a dance movement that explores three different levels. For example, 'make any movement you like that covers the ground (such as sweeping) reaches up high (such as dusting a ceiling) and involves the area between (such as polishing a table).'

2 Half the group perform these actions while the others watch. They then change over. This is followed by discussion of ways of exaggerating movement by including turning or changes of speed.

3 Individuals practise their own ideas, then half-groups demonstrate, as in stage 2.

4 Discussion of emotions experienced in everyday life: how they create tension or release it and how this affects our movements.

5 Each person is free to choose an emotion that contains tension and to use it in their dance. Practice of this is followed by half-group demonstrations as before, and then feedback.

6 Now each person chooses an emotion that releases tension and, as before, uses it in their dance. Practice, feedback and demonstration as before.

7 Group discussion of the way moods can enhance our dances, by allowing us to express our inner emotions through movement, and of the benefits of release.

8 Participants improvise a final dance incorporating both tension and release in any way they like. They demonstrate to the group.

DRAMA

Aim: To encourage looking at the role of others in certain situations from a different viewpoint
Age: Teenagers/adults
Time: 90–120 minutes
Equipment: Paper, pen

■ Activity

1   Exploration of relationship issues that have been creating tension for individuals. A list is made.

2   Clarification of the feelings that are involved: how they express themselves, internally and externally.

3   Choosing one situation from the list, discuss all the parts played by individuals within it.

4   The situation is then role-played by individuals in the group. The trainer emphasizes that they must portray it as detailed by the person whose situation it was.

5   The instigator of the situation can watch the scene the first time through, ensuring that it is an accurate representation.

6   Feedback from the group: how did they feel; did they feel as they had been told to; would they like to have changed their part in the scene and how would they have done this?

7   Everyone changes round and tries the part of another person in the scene, enacting the role in the way they feel they would in actuality. The watcher now takes part too, in their own role.

8   Feedback from the group: their feelings and any challenges or differences that were felt. The trainer explains the possibility of misinterpretations occurring when seeing things from another point of view.

9   In a final enactment, everyone plays the role they feel comfortable with in the way they feel it should be played, recognizing the importance of understanding messages from others, and the original instigator sees whether, by understanding the possibilities of other people's views, they can ease their own emotions to feel more in control.

MUSIC

Aim: To recognize the effectiveness of music as a means of enhancing relaxation

Age: Teenagers/adults

Time: One hour

Equipment: Taped music

■ Activity

1 Background music, to create a comforting environment, is playing when the participants enter the room.

2 Discussion of individuals' choices of music: what they find stimulating, what relaxes them or releases emotions.

3 Participants listen to different sorts of music provided by the trainer. Closing their eyes, they listen to the music and their own bodies to see if they can feel a release or increase of tension.

4 Feedback of feelings; clarification of the different types of music that provide stimulus and relaxation for different individuals, and the different ways that they do so.

5 Relaxation technique (sitting), using a piece of music that the group have chosen from those pieces they have listened to as the main stimulant to relaxing (no directive words from the trainer). This should last no more than five minutes.

6 Feedback.

7 Full relaxation technique (lying) — see pages 38–9 using music as the additional relaxant, as for 'Relax Down 9'.

8 Feedback and evaluation.

EXERCISE 1

Aim: To develop personal belief in physical capabilities, using imagery to enhance the concept of success
Age: Teenagers/adults
Time: Up to two hours
Equipment: Video

■ Activity

Anyone using such a workshop as this will need to be trained in this area. Only an outline of ideas to build upon is given here.

1 Warm-up routine taking at least 15 minutes.
2 Exercise-based routines used in circuits to strengthen muscle groups, or specific muscle-building exercises, according to the age of the group.
3 Building stamina by adding strength-building exercises to a circuit of timed and numbered activities.
4 Participants cool down, walking around the room, breathing slowly and deeply, but comfortably stretching their arms above heads as they do so, gradually slowing their pace and lowering their arms. The time this should take depends on the level of activity and age of participants, but as a guideline walking one to five times around the room is needed to cool down effectively.
5 A general discussion on a particular skill that each person wishes to develop. Demonstration of that skill to the group by the trainer, either personally or using a video. *Note*: within an ordinary group structure there will be many different skills that individuals wish to develop, whereas specialist groups, such as a rugby team, will wish to look at specific skills related to their sport.
6 Practice of these skills by individuals, with the trainer encouraging good practice as they do so.
7 Discussion of the benefits of mental attitude and self-belief. Participants reflect on the benefits of relaxation (see pages 38–9) then, using imagery, they focus on the following: See yourself standing in the correct position, arms, heads, shoulders correct; concentration and vision are good. See yourself preparing, making the action clear, crisp and successfully achieved. Feel good about your abilities.'
8 Feedback, discussion and evaluation.

EXERCISE 2

Aim: To encourage individuals to understand the importance of exercise for healthy living and in particular to incorporate it into their everyday lives

Age: Teenagers/adults

Time: Two to three hours

Equipment: Mats and pillows, pens, paper

■ Activity

1 The trainer makes a list of exercises that participants already do, and how often.

2 Discussion of exercise: its physical and emotional benefits (see pages 49–50).

3 The trainer stresses the importance of warming up. The group practises a simple warm-up (about 15 minutes).

4 Discussion of how participants felt before and after the warm-up (you could get them to write down their feelings before they begin and immediately afterwards).

5 The trainer emphasizes the importance of correct breathing to ensure that exercise is effective and safe.

6 Discussion of situations in which participants have noticed tiredness or lethargy and others in which they have felt full of energy. Was exercise involved? The group looks at the benefits of simple exercises throughout the day to encourage reduction of tiredness and to raise energy levels.

7 Practice of a simple exercise routine (10 minutes) using main body parts. Participants write down how they feel before they begin and when they have finished.

8 The group reflects on the more relaxed feeling that follows gentle exercise, seeing the benefits of exercise as a means of enhancing a relaxed state.

9 Practice of an exercise routine including warm-up (five minutes) main theme (10 minutes) and 'Relax Down 12' (five minutes).

EXERCISE 3

Aim: To encourage recognition that exercises can be simple, and take a short or long time
Age: Teenagers/adults
Time: Two hours
Equipment: Paper, pens

■ Activity

1   This session carries on from the previous one, identifying situations at work where lethargy or tiredness is apparent.
2   Ways of reducing these feelings (see page 52).
3   The group works out a timetable for the day that includes breaks for exercise.
4   Participants decide what form of exercise these breaks will take, such as walking up and down stairs, or standing up and stretching.
5   In pairs, participants act out situations where they sit behind a desk: how they feel, how they sit, and so on. (Body language can be looked at here.)
6   Feedback, demonstrations and discussions, looking at good and bad practice.
7   The trainer talks about simple exercise routines to use while at a desk: ankle flexes, finger and wrist manipulation, shoulder circling, stretching and breathing, and so on.
8   Participants practise these in pairs, each partner taking their turn to watch the other, making notes on changes in body language, attention span, and so on. Feedback and discussion.
9   Evaluation of the session by participants. Discussion of ways to bring about change.
10   'Relaxation 2' and Relax Down 12'.

CONTACT

Aim: To continue the process of self-awareness, by developing personal relaxation skills and looking at the use of massage

Age: Adults

Time: 90 minutes

Equipment: Mats, pillows, paper, pen

■ Activity

1 Understanding the basic concept of massage using information from professional sources.

2 Group members share experiences of any formalized massage that they have experienced.

3 The group looks at ways we soothe our bodies through touch. A list is made.

4 Individuals practise rubbing, stroking, pressing and releasing a particular part of the body, identifying likes and dislikes. They look at different pressures, light and firm touch, and review the differences.

5 Discussion of where tension is felt the most in the body. Looking at simple ways of alleviating this tension by rubbing, stroking and so on.

6 Individuals practise on themselves and then, if they consent, allow a partner to massage them. If pair work is agreed then there needs to be established the importance of the person receiving the massage stating whether they wish the masseur to use a lighter or firmer touch as the massage is taking place.

7 Group review of the session and discussion of any likes and dislikes. Exploration of the possibilities of joining an adult education class to learn massage or of going to a professional masseur.

8 'Relax Down 15'.

TENSION AND RELEASE

Aim: Individuals to leave feeling calm and in control, with the recognition that they were able to understand the difference between tension and relaxation, thereby altering the effect of the tension in their bodies

■ Activity

1 With participants lying or sitting down, use the basic relaxation technique described on pages 35–6.

2 Participants tense and release different parts of the body, starting with the feet and working up to the head. (No more than five minutes.)

3 (You can use (3) and (4) as a separate, subsequent session or continue as indicated.) Repeat (2), but this time participants do not tense; they merely aim to release the body further into its already relaxed state, moving from the feet to the head, as described on pages 38–9. The trainer tells them to focus their minds on warmth, seeing the sun, or flames from an open log fire, feeling the warmth entering their bodies and inducing a more relaxed feeling. Stay with this image for a couple of minutes.

4 Come out of the relaxation, as on page 37.

RELAX DOWN 2

BREATHING

Aim: Individuals to recognize that, by using conscious, comfortable deep breathing and picturing in their minds a previously enjoyable experience, they can enhance a relaxed state

■ Activity

1 Use the relaxation technique described on pages 38–9.

2 When participants reach their belly area, they take additional breaths that pass down through the areas that have already been relaxed, making the lower part of the body even more relaxed: for example, the trainer says," Take five deep breaths. As you breathe out, feel the warm oxygen pass through the belly, thighs, knees, calves, ankles and toes. With each breath relax deeper ... and deeper ... and deeper ..."

3 Move on to the shoulders (see page 39), the trainer says, "Take five deep breaths. As you breathe in, feel the warm air enter the body; as you breathe out, feel it pass through the shoulders, elbows, wrists and fingers. Feeling them relax ..."

4 Participants relax their heads, as described on page 39. Then they focus on the following: "a favourite place, somewhere that encourages you to feel good, such as the bath, a beach or a park. See yourself there, feel the warmth of the pleasure of being there enter your body, relaxing you and helping you to feel good, to feel happy."

5 Participants come out of the relaxation, as on page 37.

RELAX DOWN 3

GOING ON A JOURNEY

Aim: To enable participants to experience ways of enhancing a relaxed state through the use of a narration based on a journey that encourages images of comfort

■ Activity
1 Relaxing, as described on pages 38–9.
2 Having first established what people like and dislike, the trainer tells a story taking the group on a journey. For example:

"Open the curtains. The sun is shining; feel the rays encouraging you to go out. As you leave your house you begin to feel excited at the prospect of an enjoyable day. A car door opens and you enter plush, luxurious surroundings; your favourite music is playing. A cabinet opens and a drink is ready for you. You sip it gently and listen to the music as the car begins the journey. Reflect for a few moments on this wonderful feeling of being nurtured, cared for."

PAUSE

"The door opens. As you step out, you see before you the most beautiful view of valleys, lakes, woods, fields and flowers. You walk along a winding path, feeling the warmth of the sun and the cool of the breeze. You notice the wild flowers and the soft scents that waft towards you, the different colours of the leaves and the shapes of the trees. Enjoy the scene."

PAUSE

'You enter a clearing where a rustic seat awaits you. Sitting down, you take in the view, the beauty, the tranquillity of your environment. You feel good: you are content and relaxed. Enjoy this scene; feel the peace and calm enter your body."

PAUSE

"The journey home is comforting. You feel exhilarated, at peace, ready to continue with your life. As you enter your home, you say to yourself, 'I feel good. I really enjoyed today. I will do it again soon.'"

161

IMAGERY 1

Aim: Individuals recognize that they can induce a feeling of lightness in their bodies which enhances a feeling of being relaxed and secure

■ **Activity**

1   Relaxation technique described on pages 38–9.
2   The trainer encourages each individual to focus their minds, creating an image of themselves:

"Imagine you are on a bed of soft feathers or a cloud that takes all your weight. Feel the soft, floating sensation of secure weightlessness."

PAUSE

"Let yourself be taken to a park. Look down and see the activities going on. Feel secure and safe. Take yourself on a journey around the park, seeing things from different aspects."

PAUSE

"Feel safe, happy, in control, and very light. Allow yourself to be brought back again. Feel yourself being gently lowered down to your resting place. It is safe, you feel calm and in control. Begin to feel the weight enter your body, the nerve ends and muscles coming back to life. They feel calmer, more relaxed. You feel good."

3   Come out of the relaxation, as on page 37.

IMAGERY 2

Aim: To recognize the beauty of nature, its simplicity and intricacy, and the way it encourages relaxed feelings of pleasure

■ Activity

1 Participants use the relaxation technique described on pages 38–9.
2 While they focus on a favourite flower, the trainer says:

"You are planting the seed, caressing the earth around it. You are watering, then sitting back and watching as the seed grows, breaking through the earth and forming a stem."

PAUSE

"From the end of the stem comes a beautiful bud, pure, tight and secure. As you watch, it begins to unfold slowly …"

PAUSE

"The bud is opening up, changing colour and shape, creating energy, vitality, as it does so. This energy is entering your body and filling you with pleasure."

PAUSE

"The beautiful flower is in full bloom. The scent gently wafts across to you, adding to your pleasure. Watch, enjoy, relax."

PAUSE

"Evening draws in and the flower closes for the night. You both feel secure and protected, happy and content."

3 Come out of the relaxation, as on page 37.

IMAGERY 3

Aim: Through the medium of imagery, to begin to see elements of self-control, to reduce or eliminate negative physical symptoms and to learn to deal with emotional feelings that are hindering well-being

■ Activity

1   Participants relax, as described on pages 38–9, until the whole body is relaxed.
2   Use any of the following ideas to relax, creating images of:
   (a)   Seeing a negative body language and changing the way to react to it. Seeing this change the other person's body language.
   (b)   Focusing on good body language; seeing yourself using it, preventing misunderstandings.
   (c)   Seeing your worst fear before you and using challenging phrases and breathing techniques to calm yourself. Phrases such as "I can stand it" diminish the fear.
   (d)   Seeing yourself succeeding at a chore or in a situation where you fear failure.
   (e)   Seeing yourself dealing with illness and feeling "I can stand it."
   (f)   Seeing a loved one in a pleasant way in your memory, particularly after bereavement.
3   Come out of the relaxation, as on page 37.

CREATIVITY 1

Aim: To establish an individual's belief in his ability to be creative, while enhancing his feeling good, comfortable and relaxed

■ Activity

1 Use the basic relaxation technique described on pages 38–9.
2 Focusing participant's minds on a favourite object, such as a piece of furniture or china, the trainer says:

"Touch it, feel the surface, marvel at its complexity; feel the energy of its craftsmanship giving out vibrations that enter your body. Drink in the beauty of the object; enjoy it. Relax, feel content."

PAUSE

"See yourself creating such an item. Marvel at the dexterity of your hands as you create your piece."

PAUSE

"Feel the surge of pride enter your body and mind. Step back to look at the finished item. Smile. Feel good."

PAUSE

"Cover the finished item with a velvet cloth to protect it."

3 Come out of the relaxation (see page 37).

CREATIVITY 2

Aim: To recognize the beauty and warmth of colour and shape and their positive contribution to contentment, pleasure and relaxation

■ Activity

1 Use the relaxation technique described on pages 38–9.
2 Participants focus on a piece of gold, silver or crystal, resting on a cloth of velvet, as the trainer says:

"The sun shines in from a window, a ray gently consuming the gold, silver or crystal. Watch as it revolves, changing shape and colour as the sun shines on it."

PAUSE

"Feel the warmth of the rays transferring from the piece of gold, silver or crystal to you, the energy, colour and shapes creating wonderful feelings of surging vitality. Feel good, content, relaxed."

PAUSE

"The sun sinks slowly; the piece of silver, gold or crystal returns to its normal shape and colour. Slowly the light dims and the piece leaves your view."

3 Come out of the relaxation, as on page 37.

CREATIVITY 3

Aim: Individuals to recognize that they can get pleasure from an imaginary creative picture and to view other pictures as a form of recreation and relaxation

■ Activity
1 Relaxation technique, as described on pages 38–9.
2 Participants focus on an imaginary blank canvas; the trainer says:

"Choose a medium with which to paint a picture: crayons, oils, water colours, pencils, felt-tips. Create a picture or a design based on a pleasant memory of a scene or object."

PAUSE (5 minutes minimum)

"Finish it off now. Step back and admire it. Hang it on your wall, smiling as you do so and then leave the room, taking one last look as you close the door."

3 Come out of the relaxation, as on page 37.

CREATIVITY 4

Aim: Individuals to be aware of their senses of smell, touch and taste, and of the pleasure of preparing, cooking and eating something that they have made for themselves, and to be able to see eating as relaxing and not just a necessity

■ Activity

1 Participants use the relaxation technique described on pages 38–9.
2 They focus on baking a cake or cooking a meal as the trainer says:

"See yourself preparing, adding ingredients, inhaling the aromas, putting everything into a dish and watching it cook."

PAUSE

"The pleasure of a little taste as it cooks: 'perfect'."

PAUSE

"Lay it out on a plate, the aroma wafting around the room, enticing others to come and see what is cooking. Your appetite is aroused: you want to taste the finished meal."

PAUSE

"Sitting down, enjoying each delicious mouthful, the taste buds rising to the challenge, pleasure reaching every part of the body as the food is devoured. Warmth, comfort and a desire to relax engulf your body."

PAUSE

"The last mouthful: enjoy it, eating slowly. Feel content, relaxed, smile with pleasure and satisfaction."

3 Come out of the relaxation, as on page 37.

RELAX DOWN 11

MUSIC

Aim: To realize that music can help us to release tension as we listen and allow the music to enter our bodies and minds; to stimulate pleasant memories; to use music to prolong a relaxed state

■ Activity

1   Relaxation technique, as on pages 38–9.
2   As participants listen to a piece of music, the trainer says: "Listen to the rhythms and melodies; feel the sounds floating through the atmosphere, reaching your body and entering it. Feel the sounds soothe and calm you, the rhythms echoing gently, entering your body and enticing you to drift into pleasant, relaxed memories."
3   Come out of the relaxation, as on page 37.

DANCE

Aim: To kindle a desire for movement, contact and love through the medium of dance

■ Activity
The trainer can use music to enhance the state of relaxation, or just imagery.

1   After relaxing (see pages 38–9), participants focus on movement.
2   Use any of the following images:
   (a)   Seeing yourself moving to the music, loving every minute of it; moving smoothly, calmly, creatively, the pleasure relaxing you more and more deeply.
   (b)   Seeing yourself perform your dance from beginning to end. Feel good — you have expressed yourself well.
   (c)   Seeing yourself dancing with your partner or a desired partner, notice the comfort, support and warmth of the movement. Feel the pleasure and contentment enter your body as you want to dance on forever.
3   Come out of the relaxation, as on page 37.

EXERCISE

Aim: Individuals to acknowledge the skills they have in creating feelings of fitness, health and relaxation; to use these abilities to stimulate them to continue with exercise and relaxation

■ Activity
1 Participants walk around the room, consciously breathing to slow down the heart rate.
2 Occasionally they stretch their arms above their heads as they breathe in, lowering them as they breathe out.
3 They walk more slowly, breathing more deeply.
4 Smiling, feeling good, they say: "I have worked hard, I have done well."
5 Listening to their bodies, they continue to walk slowly until they feel the heart rate slowing. *Note*: With older age groups, the trainer can teach pulse taking. I do not favour this as a permanent fixture of a cool-down as I believe it can create anxiety for some individuals, but occasional use provides evidence of a person's ability to work hard and recover quickly.
6 Relaxation as described on pages 38–9, focusing on breathing and recognizing the ability of the muscles to relax further after exercise. Participants reward themselves with thoughts such as: "My body feels good, I have worked hard, I can feel the benefits"; "My muscles have stretched and feel stronger, with lots of renewed vitality"; "The calm feeling I am allowing into my body rewards it for having worked well"; "I feel good; I like being in control"; "Exercise and relaxation are good for me."
7 Come out of the relaxation, as on page 37.

RELAX DOWN 14

PHRASES

Aim: To believe in one's own ability to create and enhance a relaxed state by releasing tension and recognizing the power of the mind to deal with stress

■ Activity
1   Relaxation, as on pages 38–9.
2   Focusing on the use of phrases to enhance the relaxed state and to encourage participants to believe in their own abilities to relax themselves. For example: "Warm fresh oxygen enters my body as I breathe in"; "Stale energy leaves my body as I breathe out"; "Fresh in … stale out …"; "Energy in … tiredness out …"; "I am beginning to relax"; "I feel my body relaxing"; "The tension is leaving my body, just melting away"; "I am controlling the release of this tension"; "I am allowing my body to relax"; "I am in control"; "I feel good"; "I am relaxed".
3   Come out of the relaxation, as on page 37.

MASSAGE

Aim: Through touch, individuals to develop a desire to soothe and cherish their bodies, a major element in recognizing the importance of giving time to ourselves and enjoying it

■ Activity
1 Relaxation, as on pages 38–9.
2 The trainer says:

"Focus on an image of a person being massaged, seeing the hands move across the body, relaxing the individual as they do so."

PAUSE

"Allow that image to transfer to your body: feel the soft, manipulating, gentle strokes, caressing the body, releasing all the knots, the tensions just melting away. Feeling warm and relaxed, allow the body to comply and relax with every touch."

PAUSE

"The touch becomes lighter and lighter ... As the touch reaches your face, fingertips caress and soothe the skin as it becomes soft and relaxed."

PAUSE

"The hands finally support your head, firmly, securely, then, as they lift away, they take with them all the worries of the day, leaving you feeling calm, relaxed, refreshed, content."

3 Come out of the relaxation, as on page 37.

STABILITY ZONES AND RITUALS

Aim: Individuals to reflect on positive ways they have chosen to give themselves comfort and through this comfort to recognize the opportunity of reducing their fear of not coping

■ **Activity**

1   Relaxation, as on pages 38–9.

2   Participants focus their minds on their own ability zone and ritual which they have found creates comfort for them, as the trainer says: "See yourself there, feeling the comfort enter your body, restoring energy, calming you, releasing the tension arising from a problem. As you focus on this wonderful scene, you feel the problem melting away: it is containable, you can cope; you have done so before and you will again. You feel restored, with new energy; you can control the problem; you can deal with it."

3   Come out of the relaxation, as on page 37.

DEALING WITH AVOIDANCE

Aim: To feel able to control what have seemed uncontainable emotions, to deal with a difficult situation and feel good

■ **Activity**

1 Relaxation, as on pages 38–9.
2 Participants focus on a time when they have avoided dealing with a situation that they have described earlier. The trainer says:

"See yourself facing the person, calmly; you are in control. See yourself breathing calmly, preparing yourself to speak. Hear yourself stating your beliefs, calmly and in control."

PAUSE

"Reflect on the reaction of the other person, see their body language. Change yours to show you are in control, not aggressive or afraid. See theirs change in consequence."

PAUSE

"Feel your fear melt away, the emotions leave your body. You can cope; you are coping. It is bearable; you have made it bearable. You recognize that facing the problem is the best way to reduce fear and anxiety."

3 Come out of the relaxation, as on page 37.

THOUGHTS

Aim: To see the benefits of using realistic thoughts to challenge negative ones that previously have caused anxiety

■ **Activity**
1   Relaxation, as on pages 38–9.
2   Participants focus their minds on thoughts such as the following: "Just because I fail at something, that does not make me a complete failure"; "I do make mistakes, I do fail, but I can always learn from my failures, which turns them into a chance of success"; I have the desire not to fail, but I accept that I will at times. I can stand it"; "Failure is natural, it happens to all of us; we learn from it; that is what life is all about; no-one is perfect".
3   The group members continue, using their own phrases to encourage belief in themselves.
4   Come out of the relaxation, as on page 37.

APPENDIX

ALTERNATIVE THERAPIES

Acupuncture

This is an ancient Chinese system of medicine that restores and maintains health by the insertion of needles at precise acupuncture points, just below the body surface, in order to relieve pain and illness. The treatment itself entails inserting needles that are either withdrawn immediately or left in place for up to 20–30 minutes, and is said to stimulate endorphins which are the body's natural opiate-like painkillers, releasing tension and promoting calmness, with the ability to alter a mood from depression to optimism. Some of the many conditions that are said to be treatable with acupuncture are pain, anxiety, anger, grief, fear, diet problems, arthritis, eczema, sports injuries, hay fever, asthma, migraine, high blood pressure, menstrual disorders and intestinal problems.

If you would like further details on the use of acupuncture you can contact the British Council for Acupuncture, Park House, 206 Latimer Road, London W10 6RE on 0181-964 0222 in the UK, or, in the USA, the American Acupuncture Association, 4262 Kissena Boulevard, Flushing, New York 11344 (718-886-4431) or the American Association for Acupuncture & Oriental Medicine, 433 Front St, Catasauqua, Pennsylvania 18032 (610-266-1433).

Alexander technique

This technique bases its theory on the realignment of the body in order to remove tension and stress through relaxation practice. Its aim is to improve posture by correcting structural/postural and/or balance problems and to aid a number of medical conditions. This, practitioners believe, is achieved through creating good breathing techniques while maintaining a good posture and promoting a relaxed body position. The practice realigns the body to convert a person's negative position into a positive one which affects their physical and mental state, bringing into their consciousness previously unnoticed tension. This is achieved by working on the relationship between body parts, focusing on muscles, joints or bone alignment, and re-educating the body and mind to overcome poor habits of posture and movement, thereby reducing physical and mental tension. The main areas that practitioners work on are the head and neck and their relationship to the rest of the body. If you would like to know more, you can join one of the many adult education courses run throughout the country, or contact the Society of Teachers of the Alexander Technique, 20 London House, 266 Fulham Road, London SW10 9EL (Telephone 0171-351 0828 for further details) in the UK or, in the USA, the American Center for Alexander Technique, 129 West 67th Street, New York, New York 10023 (212-799-0468), or the North American Society of Teachers of the Alexander Technique, PO Box 517, Urbana, Illinois 61801 (217-367-6956).

Aromatherapy

This practice employs aromatic essences extracted from wild or cultivated plants for beauty treatments or therapies which are said to be similar to those used in herbal medicine. They are usually administered by massage, in baths and through inhalation, although they can also be taken internally when prescribed by medical doctors and are perceived as acting as a sedative or stimulant. It is an aromatic, health-giving treatment which uses therapeutic and pure distilled essential oils to improve the health and balance of the skin, body and mind. Practitioners encourage people to think of each plant part, even its roots and resins, as carrying an imprint or pattern of its personality and spirit, which can in turn be allowed to penetrate a person's body, using their sense of smell to produce a healing effect.

Massage is said to be the most effective way to induce essential oils into the body. This is because the stimulation and relaxation processes of the massage help the essences to penetrate the skin. The resultant improvement in circulation, which is enhanced by further gentle massage, improves the absorption and distribution of the oils' active ingredients. If you would like to know more, contact the Aromatherapy Associates, 68 Maltings Place, Bagleys Lane, Fulham, London SW6 2BY (0171-731-8129) in the UK or, in the USA, the American Phytoaromatherapy Association, 7436 Sw 117th Avenue #188, Miami, Florida 33183 (305-460-3392), or the National Association for Holistic Aromatherapy, PO Box 17622, Boulder, Colorado 80308 (415-564-6785).

Autogenic training

This is a systematized approach involving attention-focusing exercises designed to generate a state of mind and body relaxation. Some people perceive it as a form of self-hypnosis, a way of establishing self-control or healing powers that bring with them the ability to achieve deep relaxation. The word 'autogenic' means 'self-generated'. The process is therefore one in which individuals are able to relax themselves without the need of a trainer. Its main aim is to enable individuals to concentrate on their bodily sensations and breathing in order to relax the neuromuscular and vascular systems, regulating the heart rate and the breathing mechanism, creating warmth in the abdomen while cooling the forehead.

Practitioners state that, although the goals of autogenic training and of hypnosis are similar — to create sensations beginning with the warmth and heaviness of the extremities — the outcome with autogenic training is that the individual's awareness of their practice is in the awake, not trance-like, mode. If you are interested in finding out more you can contact the Centre for Autogenic Training, 101 Harley Street, London W1N 1DF (Tel 0171-935 1811) .

Bach flower remedies

Bach flower remedies derive from Dr Edward Bach, who first developed flower preparations in the 1930s, originally to treat specific emotional imbalances. For example, the 'rescue remedy' was used in emergencies to reduce the effects of trauma and encourage the body's own healing powers. Bach based the composition of his remedies on key personality types with chronic patterns of mental or emotional imbalance that created tendencies to contract certain chronic diseases, segregating his essences into single-flower bottles that could then be mixed by the practitioner to meet the needs of an individual client. The preparations are made from flower essence, the flower being immersed in water and exposed to sunlight or heat. This in turn infuses the preparation with healing properties that come from the life energy and spiritual elements that are believed to be contained within the flower. Practitioners claim that the essences strengthen the individual and allow the individual's innate spiritual powers to enhance the body's and the mind's natural healing abilities. Some counsellors use these remedies as a means of encouraging their clients to open up and explore their innermost feelings; in other words, they appear to be relaxants that encourage a 'melting away' of barriers. If you wish to know more, you can contact Dr Edward Bach Centre, Mount Vernon, Sotwell, Wallingford, Oxford OX10 0PZ (Tel 01491 834678).

Biofeedback

'Feedback' here refers to receiving information from a sensory device in order to evaluate and adjust bodily functions. Biofeedback is a process of using information obtained from various types of machines, known as relaxometers, in order to monitor and gain control over automatic, reflex-regulated body functions. The visual or auditory response of the machine makes physiological activities perceptible that we are otherwise unaware of.

It has been determined through research that there is an 'alpha state' (the most relaxed waking state) which can be achieved by an individual learning to challenge and change their state of mind. For example, chronic pain sufferers using biofeedback have been able to change not only their bodily sensitivities but also their state of mind, which has often meant seeing themselves as a whole person again. This technique has been used for, among other conditions, migraines, high blood pressure, epilepsy, pain, neck, back and shoulder injuries, and in relaxation training for childbirth. Use of this machine is often taught as part of a stress management diploma course. One such course is run by the Centre for Stress Management, 156 Westcombe Hill, Blackheath, London SE3 7DH (Tel 0181-293 4114) who will also be able to give you information on where courses are held in other parts of the UK. In the USA contact the American Applied Psychophysiology & Biofeedback Association, 10200 West 44th Avenue #304, Wheat Ridge, Colorado 80033 (303-422-8436).

Dramatherapy

As well as being used as an enhancement of dance, dramatherapy has an essence of its own that enables individuals to shed the layers of internalized emotions that create tension and anxiety, thereby inducing a more relaxed state. It is often through the creation of fiction and the entering of fictive characters that we not only understand ourselves better but are able to communicate things that otherwise we could not.

Dramatherapy workshops include the following elements: use of creative drama exercises; role-play as found in everyday life, acted out to clarify understanding of situations and behaviour as well as possible change for the future; expansion of the limits of our experiences, by stimulating our artistic and aesthetic sense; developing appropriate roles through practice and remodelling until they become natural and less conscious; encouraging personal development of different role models that are appropriate to different situations; creating new possibilities for experiencing scenes in unusual or unprescribed ways; discovering ways of connecting our internal responses with our external behaviour, and vice versa. They may also include movement, mime and improvisation, puppets and masks, sculpting, text and story work.

Homeopathy

Homeopathy was founded by Samuel Hahnemann in the early 1800s and was based on his exploration of substances that are associated with causing diseases and seeking ways of using the same substances in small doses to fight the same diseases, although the concept was mentioned by Paracelsus in the sixteenth century, when he spoke of 'substances that can make me ill but also cure me in small doses'. Homeopathic preparations or remedies are essences of naturally occurring substances derived from plants, animal materials and natural chemicals. The principle of homeopathy is that a substance which in large quantities causes illness in a healthy person can cure the same illness when it is extremely diluted. It is said by practitioners to assist the natural tendency of the body to heal itself, as they believe that all symptoms of ill health are expressions of disharmony within the whole person and that it is the *person* who needs treatment, not the disease. Many adult education courses are run as an introduction to this subject, typically involving five two-hour sessions. Sometimes a one-day course is available. These are introductory courses, comprising a personalized study of ways to recover from illness, enhance a relaxed state and reduce stress. If you would like to know more about homeopathy, contact the Society of Homeopaths, 2 Artizan Rd, Northampton NN1 4HU (01604 21400) in the UK or, in the USA, the American Institute of Homeopathy, 1585 Glencoe Street #44, Denver, Colorado 80220 (303-898-5477).

Hypnotherapy/self-hypnosis

Using the hypnotic state to heal is an ancient process that dates back to the dawn of civilization, suggestions of healing being made to a person while they were in a trance. Hypnosis is the use of suggestion to a person who passively receives ideas or instructions, allowing themselves to be receptive to them. Hypnotherapy is a process of therapy while the person is under hypnosis which is aimed at enabling them to recover from psycho-emotional traumas that are affecting their lives.

Hypnotherapy has been described by practitioners as 'the inducing of a trance-like state of heightened suggestibility or compliance. It is a state of consciousness or awareness that is not sleep but not an awake state either, where their orientation to external reality is diminished'.

Self-hypnosis is a process of self-awareness that a person is encouraged to use during times of stress in order to produce within themselves a relaxed and altered state, free from anxiety. In order to achieve this, it is recognized that a person needs an open mind, together with genuine motivation to change the way they feel, with the time to do so in a quiet place with the aid of effective (for them) hypnotic suggestions.

Examples of this trance-like state occur when we daydream, or when deep relaxation is achieved. It is important to recognize that emotional distress can also induce this state. If you wish to know more, you can contact either the British Society of Hypnotherapy, on 0171-385 1166, or the Association of Curative Hypnotherapists, 8 Balaclava Rd, Kings Heath, Birmingham B14 7SG (0121-441-1775), in the UK or, in the USA, the American Hypnotherapy Association, 18607 Ventura Boulevard #310, Tarzana, California 91356 (818-344-4464).

Massage

Massage derives its name from a Greek word meaning to knead. It is a systematic approach which uses therapeutic stroking and kneading that is applied to the soft tissues of the body to produce beneficial effects in the nervous system, circulation, muscles and ligaments by relaxing the body and mind. It is a sensual healing art that is claimed by practitioners to reduce emotional tension and anxiety, replacing it with a feeling of calm and trust, symbolizing caring, friendship, affection and tenderness. A session is said to stimulate or sedate, depending on the nature or style of the strokes applied. You can find out more by contacting the College of Massage, 5 Newman Passage, London W1P 3PF (0171-637 7125) in the UK or, in the USA, the American Massage Therapy Association, 820 Davis Street #100, Evanston, Illinois 60201 (708-864-0123).

Meditation

The word 'meditation' comes from a Sanskrit word for wisdom, so when we meditate we are said to be increasing our wisdom. Meditation is seen as a means of reaching that part inside us that contains our internal information, so by turning inwards we are able to gain an insight into ourselves. It is practised in a comfortable position, in a quiet environment, using controlled breathing. The aim, according to practitioners, is to be able to adopt a physically relaxed and mentally passive attitude while channelling thoughts onto a single object. There can be many variations of this object to allow for the individual needs of a person and to ensure 'comfort' with it, such as image, happening, thought repetition, a word or phrase said out loud (as in mantra meditation) or breathing rhythms. The ultimate aim is to learn the discipline of concentration (focus) on only one aspect at a time, not allowing the mind to wander, and if it does wander to bring it back, so that by delving into what we experience we can help ourselves to find the solution of a possible problem. Practitioners say the outcome is to combat self-destructive thoughts by focusing on the positive until that belief becomes part of a person's make-up.

If you would like to know about the skills of a meditation trainer you can contact the School of Meditation, 158 Holland Park Avenue, London W11 4UR (0171-603 6116).

Reflexology

This is the application of controlled pressure by thumb and index finger to the reflex points of the feet, for example, to release tension, often perceived as a therapeutic massage. It is believed that, by applying pressure to one part of the body, you can effect changes in another part, recognizing that, as muscles relax, there is a stimulation of the body's natural ability to heal itself. Reflexology can be traced back to Chinese medical philosophy and theory as an energy meridian.

Practitioners use the soles of the feet and the palms of the hands as maps of the whole body. They believe that by massaging these extremities they are able to send messages to different areas of the body that stimulate reflexes and nerve impulses. This they say loosens bodily tensions and enables energy to flow freely, stimulating the blood circulation to nourish the body and the lymph system to cleanse it, encouraging sluggish glands and organs to regain normal functioning.

The technique itself tends to be broken down into hand reflexology, foot reflexology, zone therapy and body reflexology and is often used by practitioners alongside massage, so that an overall state of bodily relaxation is achieved. Its benefits are that it is simple, easy to learn as a self-help mechanism and encourages empathic contact with a friend or partner. If you are interested in this technique you can join one of the many adult education classes that are available, or contact the British Reflexology Association.

T'ai-chi-ch'uan

This is said to date from fourteenth-century China, where it was recognized that anxiety, irritation and fear, by causing tension, can also cause disease by interfering with breathing and circulation and the general functioning of the body. It is one of many martial arts that have a foundation in ancient Chinese rituals, where movement is seen as descriptive but also as a relaxant, advocated as a means of eliminating stress-related diseases. Practitioners claim that it calms both body and mind, relieving stress and anxiety, deepening breathing capacity and so improving organs that function better with the use of fresh oxygen. The technique itself aims to centre on relaxing the whole body by deepening breathing, to improve co-ordination, to loosen joints, increase flexibility and encourage self-control through patience and perseverance, with practice improving muscle tone and self-understanding as well as cultivating poise and a calm spirit. This Chinese form of gentle and relaxing exercise is performed with smoothly flowing movements in a sequence. It originally consisted of 128 relaxed held postures, flowing one into another without a break. Now it has between 35 and 50 movements that can take up to 10 minutes to perform.

It is available as a class format in adult education colleges, or you can contact the British T'ai Chi Ch'uan Association, on 0171-935 8444, for more information and advice on books to read. In the USA contact the Tai Chi Chuan/Shaolin Chuan Association, 33W614 Roosevelt Road, PO Box 430, Geneva, Illinois 60134 (708-232-0029).

Yoga

This is a movement-based exercise regime that focuses on breathing and stretching the body into held positions; there is also a relaxation component to enhance the overall feeling of restored energy. The aim is for the individual to achieve a heightened personal degree of physical, mental and spiritual unison, by improving suppleness, posture, breathing and strength, as well as general fitness.

Yoga focuses on a series of static or stretching exercises linked with breathing and the ability of the mind to meditate and achieve a calm, relaxed state, even while holding a position where a muscle is stretched. This is because a stretched muscle reduces the tension held within and can then relax into the stretch, creating stillness, then comfort, and through this a relaxed state. The purpose of the meditation is to enhance a person's ability to observe physiological functions and the way they are connected to their emotional states and reactions.

Yoga is seen as an essential way of learning to look after yourself and is quite widely practised by individuals and groups in the Western Hemisphere. There are several styles, but the most widely used is Hatha or Iyengar; certainly this has been the case in adult education in Britain, where at one time there were as many as 18 classes a week in one borough alone. If you would like to know more, you can contact the Iyengar Yoga Institute, 223a Randolph Avenue, London W9 1NL (0171-624 3080), or the Yoga for Health Foundation, on 0171-672-7271 in the UK or, in the USA, the American Yoga Association, 513 South Orange Avenue, Sarasota, Florida 34236 (813-953-5859).

BIBLIOGRAPHY

Atkinson JM, *Coping with Stress at Work*, Thorsons, 1988.
Benson H, *The Relaxation Response*, Collins, 1976.
British Acupuncture Association Handbook, 1995.
British Medical Association, *Complementary Medicine*, 1993.
Brown B, *Stress and the Art of Biofeedback*, Harper & Row, 1977.
Burns D, *The Feeling Good Handbook*, Plume, 1990.
Campbell J, *Creative Art in Groupwork*, Winslow Press, 1993.
Carroll S & Smith T, *Complete Family Guide to Healthy Living*,
  Dorling Kindersley, 1992.
Chaitow L, *The Stress Protection Plan*, Thorsons, 1992.
Cheney G & Strader J, *Modern Dance*, Allyn & Bacon, 1977.
Cooper CL, Cooper RD & Eaker LH, *Living with Stress*,
  Penguin, 1988.
Coxhead N, *Mind Power*, Unwin, 1987.
Downing G, *The Massage Book*, Penguin, 1974.
Dyke P & Dyke C, *Relaxation in a Week*, Hodder & Stoughton,
  1992.
Hastings J, *You Can Have What You Want*, Touchstone, date
  unknown.
Heron C, *The Relaxation Therapy Manual*, Winslow, 1996.
Hodgkinson L, *How It Can Help You*, Piatkus, 1988.
Homeopathy: the Family Handbook, Thorsons, 1992.
Inkeles G, *Super Massage*, Piatkus, 1988.
Iyengar BKS, *The Concise Light on Yoga*, Unwin, 1980.
Jennings S, *Creative Drama in Groupwork*, Winslow Press, 1986.
Karlins M & Andrews LM, *Turning on the Power of Your Mind*,
  Warner Paperback, 1973.
Kaye A & Matcham DC, *Reflexology*, Thorsons, 1978.
Lawrence R, *Journey into Supermind*, Souvenir Press, 1995 (out
  of print).
Lever R, *Hypnotherapy for Everyone*, Penguin, 1988.
Levete G, *No Handicap to Dance*, Souvenir Press, 1982.
Lindenfield G, *Assert Yourself*, Thorsons, 1986.
Madder J, *Relax and Be Happy*, Unwin, 1987.

Markham U, *Hypnosis*, Macdonald Optima, 1987.

Maxwell-Hudson C, *Complete Book of Massage*, Dorling Kindersley, 1990.

McIntyre M, *Herbal Medicine for Everyone*, Penguin, 1988.

Mindell E, *The Vitamin Bible*, Arlington Books, 1992.

Mitchell L, *Simple Relaxation*, Murray, 1988.

Norman L, *Reflexology Handbook*, Thomas Caron – Piatkus, 1988.

Olsen K, *Alternative Health Care*, Piatkus, 1991.

Palmer S, *Stress Management Course Reader*, Centre for Stress Management, 1992.

Palmer S & Dryden W, *Counselling for Stress Problems*, Sage, 1995.

Payne H, *Creative Movement & Dance in Groupwork*, Winslow Press, 1990.

Powell K, *Fight Stress and Win*, Thorsons, 1988.

Price S, *Practical Aromatherapy*, Thorsons, 1983.

Proto L, *Meditation for Everybody*, Penguin, 1991.

Proto L, *Total Relaxation*, Penguin, 1991.

Schaffer M, *Bach Flower Therapy Theory & Practise*, Thorsons, 1986.

Simonton OC, Simonton SM & Creighton JL, *Getting Well Again*, Bantam, 1991.

Smith T, *Understanding Homeopathy*, Insight, 1987.

Stevens C, *Alexander Technique*, Macdonald Optima, 1987.

The Holistic Network Directory (available in libraries).

Tisserand M, *Aromatherapy for Women*, Thorsons, 1985.

Ullman D, *Homeopathy Medicine for the 21st Century*, Thorsons, 1989.

Understanding Stress, Which? Consumer Guide, 1988.

AUDIO-VISUAL AIDS

There are many audio-visual aids you can borrow, hire or buy, to use in your workshops, available from stationers, Health Authority resource centres and adult education colleges. These include health charts on all areas of health awareness for all ages; 'healthy living' handouts, available from health authorities and supermarkets. The media resources departments of adult education colleges will provide advice on how to make your own visual aids, while the contacts suggested for alternative therapies (see pages 179–186) will also be of assistance. Age Concern provides help with audio-visual aids for elderly people.

As the use of sound is very much dependent on the likes and dislikes of particular individuals, you can establish what works for you and your clients by borrowing records or cassettes from your local library (sometimes only available in the main branch). When you feel confident about your requirements there are many music shops, stationers and direct suppliers who can provide the aids you need. For example, Winslow provide a complete library of music for relaxation, including natural sounds and relaxation videos and cassettes. You can contact them on 01869 244733.

ALPHABETICAL LIST OF ACTIVITIES

Also in the Creative Activity Series ...

This unique series' common theme is to provide creative activity ideas for use with groups of all ages.

Creative Action Methods in Groupwork

Andy Hickson

Highly practical and accessible, with emphasis on participative groupwork and good working practices, this unique manual outlines action method techniques for exploring difficulties and problems.

Creative Writing in Groupwork

Robin Dynes

Here are over 100 stimulating activities designed to help participants express themselves, explore situations, compare ideas and develop both imagination and creative ability.

Creative Drama in Groupwork

Sue Jennings

150 ideas for drama in this completely practical manual make it a veritable treasure trove which will inspire everyone to run drama sessions creatively, enjoyably and effectively.

Creative Movement & Dance in Groupwork

Helen Payne

This innovative book explores the link between movement and emotion and provides 180 activities and ideas for the use of dance movement to enrich therapy and programmes.

Creative Art in Groupwork

Jean Campbell

Highly accessible, this manual contains 142 art activities developed for use with groups of people of all ages.

Creative Relaxation in Groupwork

Irene Tubbs

Offering a goldmine of techniques and processes, this essential text provides more than 100 practical ideas for groups that need to work on relaxation.

For further information or a free catalogue, please contact:

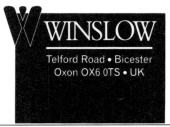

WINSLOW

Telford Road • Bicester
Oxon OX6 0TS • UK